Experiential Unity
Theory and Model

Experiential Unity Theory and Model

Treating Trauma in Therapy

Alyson Quinn

Second Edition

LEXINGTON BOOKS
Lanham • Boulder • New York • London

Published by Lexington Books
An imprint of The Rowman & Littlefield Publishing Group, Inc.
4501 Forbes Boulevard, Suite 200, Lanham, Maryland 20706
www.rowman.com

86-90 Paul Street, London EC2A 4NE

British Library Cataloguing in Publication Information Available

Library of Congress Cataloging-in-Publication Data

Names: Quinn, Alyson, 1959- author.
Title: Experiential unity theory and model : treating trauma in therapy / Alyson Quinn.
Description: Second edition. | Lanham : Lexington Books, [2022] | Includes
    bibliographical references and index. | Summary: "The second edition of Experiential
    Unity Theory and Model: Treating Trauma in Therapy addresses the current concerns
    dominating the field of group therapy and individual counseling and promotes a
    healing milieu whereby clients can address the core of their problems and heal
    fully"—Provided by publisher.
Identifiers: LCCN 2022003067 (print) | LCCN 2022003068 (ebook) |
    ISBN 9781793648648 (hardcover) | ISBN 9781793648655 (epub)
Subjects: LCSH: Experiential psychotherapy. | Group psychotherapy. | Group
    counseling.
Classification: LCC RC489.E96 Q85 2022 (print) | LCC RC489.E96 (ebook) |
    DDC 616.89/152--dc23/eng/20220315
LC record available at https://lccn.loc.gov/2022003067
LC ebook record available at https://lccn.loc.gov/2022003068

To my parents Stanley and Elaine Quinn—your fierce curiosity and openness to healing modalities all around the globe flung open doors for me and propelled me to develop Experiential Unity model.

Contents

List of Figures

Acknowledgments

First, I would like to thank the staff at Lexington Books, especially Kasey Beduhn for her help and guidance along the way. Enormous gratitude to Yvonne Haist who painstakingly waded through the manuscript and provided a thorough scholarly review shining the light on gaps in the text. Special thanks to Brooke Kelly, a dedicated illustrator, who crafted the images by immersing herself in the metaphor bringing them to life in their final form. Thanks also to Jonas Baltakis for his immense skill in helping with the bibliography. Thank you too for all the clients I have worked with over the years whose intense struggle helped me to dig deeper to discover "what works" in the healing process. Lastly, to my family and friends—am ever grateful for your love and support.

Chapter 1

Brief Trauma History and Influence of Neuroscience

The earliest writings of trauma and its impact on the human condition were recorded on cuneiform tablets from ancient Sumer over 4,000 years ago. Citizens' reactions to the death of their king Urnamma were described in symptoms which revealed ongoing sleep and mood disturbances.

Herodotus, a renowned Greek author in 440 BCE, also wrote about trauma reactions from accounts of war. He describes the impact of witnessing the death of another soldier as being "stricken with blindness" (Figley, Ellis, Reuther, & Gold, 2017, p. 1) even though there were no personal injuries suffered. These earlier understandings of psychological trauma did not consolidate into a theory until the mid- to late nineteenth century. Up until that point, trauma was focused on physical wounds and trauma to the entire body; this definition remains in place—for example, hospital systems have trauma units and specialists focusing on trauma care.

The historical roots of modern-day trauma care link back to the 1860s with an understanding of the impact of "shock," which was termed at the time as the "wounding of the mind brought about by sudden, unexpected, emotional shock" (Figley, Ellis, Reuther, & Gold, 2017, p. 4). Jean-Martin Charcot, considered the father of both modern neurology and psychiatry in France, made a significant contribution to understanding trauma with his work on patients with hysteria. He emphasized the concept of mental factors in hysteria and his work influenced many at the time, including Sigmund Freud. Freud (1962), in his paper "The Aetiology of Hysteria" (1896/1962), posited that when symptoms remained after addressing the original event it could be that an earlier, more significant and likely repressed experience, could be contributing to the symptomology.

A deeper understanding of trauma was also derived from "railway spine" syndrome. *Railway spine syndrome* refers to the range of symptoms individuals experienced after a railway accident, even though they had no physical injuries. The range of symptoms could include restlessness, helplessness, and other somatic issues. Many suggest this was an early understanding of the concept of posttraumatic stress disorder, as it challenged the assumptions of medicine at the time that any injury needed a known physiological manifestation. This undercurrent of suspiciousness and judgment regarding illness that has no physical signs and symptoms has contributed a great deal to the pathologizing of those experiencing trauma. Assumptions in the medical field at the time was that "there had to be a known and discernable physiological cause; otherwise, such complaints were considered tantamount to malingering or feigning" (Figley, Ellis, Reuther, & Gold, 2017, p. 4).

The experiences of war continued to impact assumptions and diagnoses, and soldier's experiences challenged the belief that all symptoms had to be rooted in a physical ailment. Although *shell shock* was a term coined at the time that helped explain the variety of somatic experiences such as hyperarousal, amnesia, and other psychological experiences, it was deemed to be a result of cerebral hemorrhaging or micro-lesions in the brain and spinal cord.

In the late nineteenth century, a significant shift occurred and many "practitioners began to reject and transcend reliance on a wholly physical explanation, especially in the absence of evidence of physical injuries" (Figley, Ellis, Reuther, & Gold, 2017, p. 5).

War and its psychological impact continued to challenge restrictive diagnoses. The first term that described the concept of trauma was *Gross stress reaction* (GSR) under the Diagnostic and Statistical Manual of Mental Disorders (DSM) (American Psychiatric Association, 1952). The diagnosis specifically addressed trauma related to combat and other major disasters. "A particularly important feature of GSR was that it was explicitly recognized to be a reaction to an event, rather than an expression of an inborn defect or vulnerability" (Figley, Ellis, Reuther, & Gold, 2017, p. 5).

Soldiers returning from the Vietnam War, with a wide range of symptomology, created more pressure on the field to study and legitimize their experiences. An initial term coined at the time was *post-Vietnam syndrome*. Eventually in 1980 a PTSD diagnosis was included in the DSM III; this finally legitimized the concept of trauma and its impact on the individual. Initially the term *trauma* referred to an experience that was "beyond ordinary human experience" (cited in Figley, Ellis, Reuther, & Gold, 2017, p. 5). Later DSM's manuals broadened this idea to include reactions to the event—it could include a range of emotions such as "intense fear, helplessness and horror" (cited in Figley, Ellis, Reuther, & Gold, 2017, p. 5).

In the 1970s, alongside the shifts in treating those with trauma symptoms, other discoveries were also contributing to an overall understanding of human behavior and traumatic memory. Dr. Candace Pert, a neuro-pharmacologist and titled the "Goddess of Neuroscience," provided scientific evidence through her research that impacted our understanding of emotions. She stated, "the chemicals that are running our body and brain are the same chemicals that are involved in emotion. And that says to me we better pay more attention to emotions with respect to our health" (Chatfield, n.d.). Her ideas at the time were a radical shift for Western medicine and helped to challenge current ethos and promote an understanding that the mind and body were interconnected, and that the body was in fact the subconscious mind. This had been long accepted by Ayurvedic medicine, Chinese medicine, and some indigenous cultures from around the world. By contrast, Rene Descartes significantly reinforced the mind/body disconnection. He needed human bodies for dissection and so he promised the church "Anything to do with the soul, mind, or emotions, I leave to the clergy. I will only claim the realm of the body" (Figley, Ellis, Reuther, & Gold, 2017, p. 3). This has historically been referred to the Cartesian split where the mind and body were separate entities and its ideas still permeate modern medicine, with emotional concerns at times labeled psychosomatic or relegated to the psychiatric domain.

Pert also contributed to ideas about trauma, with specific attention to feelings. She purported a notion that is held by neuroscience regarding embodied emotion:

> I believe all emotions are healthy, because emotions are what unite the mind and the body. Anger, fear, sadness, the so-called negative emotions, are as healthy as peace, courage, and joy. To repress these emotions and not let them flow freely is to set up a dis-integrity in the system, causing it to act at cross-purposes rather than as a unified whole. The stress this creates, which takes the form of blockages and insufficient flow of peptide signals to maintain function at the cellular level, is what sets up the weakened conditions that can lead to disease."(Chatfield, n.d.)

She also recommended in her outlined eight-part Program, "get in touch with your body. Your body is your subconscious mind, and you can't heal it by talk alone. We can access our minds and our emotions through the physical body. Use bodywork or movement therapy to heal stuck emotions" (Chatfield, n.d.).

Along with Candace Pert, other neuroscientists and scientists from the field of cognitive science continued to influence the counseling field and an understanding of the impact of trauma. For example, neuroscience and neuroimaging assist the field by measuring structural changes in the brain due to the impact of counseling. For both counseling and trauma work five principles in neuroscience are highly relevant. An article adapted from

Intentional Interviewing and Counseling: Facilitating Client Development in a Multicultural Society, 7th edition, Allen Ivey, Mary Bradford Ivey, and Carlos Zalaquett (2013), highlights the following key areas:

- Neuroplasticity—It is the lifelong capacity of the brain to create new brain cells and new neural pathways. This is key to the healing of trauma as it assists the client in rewiring learned responses to life's stressors.
- Neurogenesis—It is the process by which new neurons are formed in the brain. It impacts several areas of the brain and can assist in creating new neural networks.
- Attention and focus—Factors involved in attention and focus include arousal which engages the reticular activating system at the brain's core. This process transmits stimuli to the cortex and activates neurons to fire in many regions of the brain.
- Clarifying and understanding emotions—It is common for people to have a limited vocabulary when describing how they feel. Paying attention to the specificity of feeling is key as different feelings fire up different parts of the brain. A term called *granularity of emotion* refers to the ability to detect finer grained emotions. According to neuroscientist Lisa Feldman Barrett those people with "higher emotional granularity go to the doctor less frequently, use medication less frequently, and spend fewer days hospitalized for illness" (Barrett, 2016).
- Focusing on wellness and positives—according to research an effective executive frontal cortex focusing on positives and strengths can assist in overcoming negative consequences.

Another important development for understanding the impact of trauma was the FMRI, a technique that measured brain activity. It was developed by Seiji Ogawa, Kâmil Uğurbil, and Ken Kwong (2012). This made a significant contribution to neuroscience and became a popular tool for imaging normal brain function—especially for psychologists. Over the last decade it has provided new insight into how memories are formed and insights into language, pain, learning, and emotion to name a few areas of research. Some studies have researched participant's ability to control emotion, which helps to inform future therapeutic applications.

Both neuroimaging and biochemical advances have helped to clarify the biological impact of trauma. The new insights include the following areas:

1) Trauma disrupts homeostasis and can have a short or long-term impact on both biological systems and a variety of organs.
2) According to Van der Kolk, trauma influences the way children organize and process information and what they may imagine in their future and their present focus (Van der Kolk, 2015).

3) Trauma influences the way threat is perceived from a feeling, behavior, and thinking perspective and workings of the biological systems.
4) Trauma impacts the biological processes in attachment and the infant's limbic system, which impacts their ability to adapt to changing circumstances.
5) According to Schore, "There is now agreement that, in general, the enduring effects of traumatic abuse are due to deviations in the development of patterns of social information processing. I suggest that, in particular, early trauma alters the development of the right brain, the hemisphere that is specialized for the processing of socioemotional information and bodily states" (Schore, 2001, p. 9).

Allan Schore, considered a world leader in Attachment theory and known as the "American Bowlby," was among the first to consolidate the latest brain science on how an infant's brain forms biologically (developmental neuroscience) with the early psychology of the infant mind (developmental psychoanalysis). Schore, alongside other somatically oriented professionals, has made a significant contribution to in advancing the field pertaining to the understanding of trauma, its impact, and treatment methods. Allan Schore's research additionally focused on self-regulation; it emphasizes the importance of paying attention to subtle body signs. In the last couple of decades, particularly the last 10 years, there have been other notable contributions that have added substantially to an understanding of the role of the body in healing the mind. They include Alan Fogel and his research on the "felt sense," in 2009, which increased an understanding of embodied self-awareness. Another key contributor to a trauma-informed approach is Stephen Porges and his research, since 1994, on Polyvagal theory. Polyvagal theory is an amalgamation of evolutionary, neuroscientific, and psychological theories that focuses on the role of the vagus nerve in relation to a fear response, and its capacity to attune to social cues and emotional regulation.

Polyvagal Theory provides a physiological and psychological understanding of how and why clients move through a continual cycle of mobilization, disconnection and engagement. Through the lens of Polyvagal Theory, we see the role of the autonomic nervous system as it shapes clients' experiences of safety and affects their ability for connection. (Dana, 2018, p. xvii)

A further important addition to understanding trauma is the Window of Tolerance, first coined by Daniel Siegel in 1999; it described the levels of both psychological and physiological arousal. The window is the middle zone between hypoarousal and hyperarousal. Peter Levine has also been a major contributor to trauma-informed work. His model Somatic Experiencing has been instrumental in how to work somatically, and he has incorporated concepts such as titration and pendulation to explain the careful pacing needed when working through trauma. Levine states that

> In renegotiating trauma via Somatic Experiencing we utilize "pendulation," the shifting of body sensations or emotions between those of expansion and those of contraction. This ebb and flow allows the polarities to gradually be integrated. It is the holding together of these polarities that facilitates deep integration and often an "alchemical," transformation. (Ross, 2018)

Pat Ogden, founder of Sensorimotor Psychotherapy, in her book written by her and her colleagues, *Trauma and the Body* (2006), describes a model of working through trauma that integrates three realms of experience, namely somatic, cognitive, and emotional. Sensorimotor psychotherapy is a body-oriented approach and it places emphasis on the somatic dimension to gain access to memories that are encoded as sensory fragments or physical patterns. It draws on a wide range of theoretical underpinnings including Polyvagal theory, interpersonal neurobiology, attachment, affect regulation theory, and structural disassociation. Another major contribution to the field of understanding trauma and its impact has been the work of Bessel Van de Kolk. He has emerged as a leader with both research and his publications, particularly his seminal work *The Body Keeps the Score* (2015). The American College of Psychotherapy describes his contribution as "There are many who change how others think, but few with the wisdom and courage, to influence the path of an entire professional culture. Such a man is Bessel Van der Kolk" (Hulon, W. American college of Psychotherapy website, 2018).

Another critical development advancing the field is an increased understanding of how trauma impacts racialized communities and individuals. Terms such as intergenerational or multigenerational trauma and historical, collective, and race-based trauma focus on these aspects. From the critical race theory (CRT) perspective, it is critical to move "beyond a color-blind framework to talking explicitly about race and, ultimately, acknowledging racism as a trauma itself is one of the first steps in trauma-informed practice from a CRT lens" (Quiros, Varghese & Vanidestine, 2019, p. 9). Many clients, or their families of origin, have experienced the terror and ravages of colonization, slavery, structural oppression, food insecurity, war, emotional and sexual violations, violence at home, and structural discrimination based on class, race, gender, and sexual orientation to name some of the societal structures and family trauma that have impacted people and left a long line of intergenerational trauma.

> Anti-oppressive practices, like other forms of social justice-oriented practice, are lenses for viewing the world, ways of asking questions and techniques for

reaffirming social justice-oriented social workers' commitment to resist, expand resources to the oppressed, redistribute power and resist again in the new spaces and opportunities that open up as a result of that resistance." (Mullaly & West, 2018, p. 291)

Clinical work with racialized individuals and communities needs a commitment to an ongoing reflection on Whiteness, a commitment to a decolonizing lens, and an anti-oppressive practice. The following are some factors to take into consideration:

- Redistribution of power in clinical practice—this aligns with a trauma-informed practice with an emphasis on bottom-up processing. In this orientation the clinician views the client as the expert on their somatic experience and the socio-cultural context of their present situation, including cultural determinants. The clinician role models cultural humility and a willingness to walk alongside the client experiencing trauma.
- Conscientization of the clinician occurs through an ongoing process of deconstruction of historical and current sociopolitical contexts. This includes a commitment to systemic focused interrogation, examining systems, reflections on Whiteness, policies, and procedures impacting the client and their community.
- A right-to-right brain orientation, critical to trauma engagement and sensory information, is a way of collaborating from an anti-colonial positionality. With an emphasis on sensations, images, tensions, and surfacing memory in the body the client is able to unpack and honor the truth of "what happened" and how they experienced the traumatic situation. This way of working protects the client from an impositional framework interpreting their experience or prescribing a model from the top-down.
- An orientation toward resistance, resilience, and a strength-based focus on "what happened." The clinician is highlighting counter-narratives that challenge the existing dominant culture and pathologizing narrative of "what's wrong with you" and unhelpful labels.
- Privileging indigenous ways of healing is a key commitment to a decolonizing practice. "In communities with histories of marginalization, the active (if unintentional) marginalization of their worldviews and ways of healing within the counseling process itself represents another form of oppression and possible trauma instead of a form of healing from trauma" (Goodman, 2015, p. 66).
- Engaging in participatory action research. "The counseling profession has an opportunity to decolonize our understanding and definitions of counseling competence through collaborative engagement with our clients in the research process. The multicultural counseling movement was

founded on the assumption that many clients were being treated unjustly within traditional, universal models of counseling practice" (Goodman, 2015, p. 51).

Given the dramatic changes in the understanding of trauma and its impact new professional designations have emerged that integrate findings of neuroscience into professional specialty areas. For instance, *Neurocounseling* is defined as "the integration of neuroscience into the practice of counseling, by teaching and illustrating the physiological underpinnings of many of our mental health concerns" (Field, Jones, & Russell-Chapin, 2017, p. 93). A neuropsychologist is someone who specializes in understanding the brain and behavior. A neuropsychiatrist diagnoses and treats behavioral and mental disorders caused by conditions affecting the nervous system, such as head injuries, epilepsy, dementia, or obsessive-compulsive disorder.

Chapter 2

Experiential Unity Model (Group and Individual) and Therapy Informed by Neuroscience for Trauma

Experiential Unity model was devised in 2010 as a way of engaging clients in a group therapy program in deeper work and to assist clients with trauma. It was later developed into both a group therapy and individual therapy model. Lately it has also been utilized in couple's counseling.

Group therapy in an institutional setting often has a strong psycho-educational focus. For instance, a client may attend a program for a concern with intense depression or anxiety symptoms, and is then enlisted in a coping with depression or anxiety group to help reduce their symptomology. From a trauma-informed perspective, the symptoms of depression and anxiety may be a direct result of trauma; therefore if the trauma is untreated, the symptoms may re-appear later. The "revolving door" aspect of client treatment—for instance, the client appears to benefit from group therapy only to experience an increase in symptoms soon after discharge—was the initial impetus for developing Experiential Unity model. The models often utilized in group therapy programs in Vancouver, Canada are cognitive behavioral therapy (CBT) or a dialectical behavioral therapy (DBT). An alternative treatment modality offered is a psychodynamic group. In psychodynamic groups the focus is on client interactions in the "here and now" and insight into their ways of relating with others. According to Yalom and Crouch (1990), an existential psychiatrist and a group psychotherapist insight is categorized into four different levels:

- How others see the patient
- What the patient is doing in relation to others
- Why the patient may be doing what he/she is doing in relationship to others
- Genetic insights.

Experiential Unity model is an integrative model and includes both insight-oriented material based on the clients' somatic experience and the "here and now" experiential component. It also includes a wide range of techniques to engage the mind and body for both group and individual therapy formats. It uses metaphor, as a right brain orientation, to bypass the conscious mind and elicit material from unconscious processes. According to Wise and Nash, "Engaging metaphor as the mediator between the devastating sensorial bodily memory of trauma and the explicit verbal narrative of what happened allows opportunities for bridging between fragmented parts of the self to occur" (Wise & Nash, 2013, p. 99).

Experiential Unity model for both Individual and Group therapy aligns with the following principles informed by neuroscience for the treatment of trauma:

- Right-to-right brain orientation of the clinician and the client
- Bottom-up processing
- Focus on implicit memory
- Ongoing tracking of arousal within the window of tolerance
- Focus on experiential work
- Incorporation of mindfulness and integrative techniques to engage the body, and process unintegrated emotions and experiences that have not been metabolized by the body. Some of the techniques include breathing, tapping, Kundalini yoga, visualizations, and mindfulness.

Additionally, Experiential Unity model engages right mode-mediated somatic work supported by Stephen Porges's Polyvagal theory. Three key principles underlie Polyvagal theory: hierarchy, neuroception, and co-regulation. These key principles are utilized in Experiential Unity model in the moment-to-moment tracking of psychobiological processes.

Hierarchy refers to the three pathways the autonomic nervous system responds to in relation to signals from the external world and body sensation. "The three pathways (and their patterns of response), in revolutionary order from the oldest to the newest, are the dorsal vagus (immobilization), the sympathetic nervous system (mobilization), and the ventral vagus (social engagement and connection)" (Dana, 2018, p. 4). On a moment-by-moment basis the autonomic nervous system is responding most often below conscious awareness and is in constant flux in reaction to others in the environment—the cues can invite regulation or an increase in reactivity. In therapeutic engagement, there is an opportunity for connection, but the ongoing tracking of the autonomic nervous system's response to the somatic work is critical. Experiential Unity model, like other integrative models, tracks the psycho-physiological processes to understand the clients' reactions to the therapeutic engagement and to their present situation. For example, a client may want desperately to connect with the therapist and share their current concerns, but their body may feel unsafe given their history of violations and so they may automatically move into a dysregulated state and may find it challenging to be in the room. The therapist from an Experiential Unity model perspective tracks reactivity and focuses on resourcing the client when dysregulation is observed.

Other key components of Polyvagal theory include neuroception and co-regulation. Neuroception, considered detection without awareness, is a key component in therapeutic trauma work. According to Dana,

> trauma trained therapists are taught that a foundation of effective work is understanding "perception is more important than reality." Personal perception, not the actual facts of an experience creates posttraumatic consequences. Polyvagal theory demonstrates that even before the brain makes meaning of an incident, the autonomic nervous system has assessed the environment and initiated an adaptative survival response. Neuroception precedes perception. (Dana, 2018, p. 6)

In Experiential Unity model, both Individual and Group sessions commence with mindfulness, breathwork, and other integrative techniques to assist the client connect with deeper processes. Exploring "sensation in the body as a way of knowing" is key as the client's body is revealing how the person is perceiving their present moment experience, also noting micro movements which reveal unconscious reactions and perceptions. Dr. Porges "coined the term neuroception to describe the way our autonomic nervous system scans for cues of safety, danger, and life threat without involving the thinking parts of the brain" (Dana, 2018. p. 8).

Co-regulation is another key factor in Experiential Unity model in both Individual and Group therapy formats. The therapeutic relationship and the attunement to the client is a key component of the healing process. In a group setting Experiential Unity model uses a bottom-up processing structure, which encourages the clients to take an active role in their healing and also in creating a healing milieu for others to co-regulate. For example, clients give each other feedback on strengths after an individual completes a "check-in"; this helps to establish trust and a sense of safety early on in the group and assists in the process of relationally regulating one another.

Experiential Unity model individual sessions all commence with mindfulness, breath-work, visualizations, or another calming technique practiced by both the clinician and client. This assists in the mutual attunement and co-regulation process as well as the capacity of the clinician to "be present" to the clients' somatic experience. Bonnie Badenoch describes the importance of the process of co-regulation thus: "we are foundationally and eternally attaching beings whose neural circuitry is open to the nourishing, co-regulating influence of others who can offer us a safe, non-judgemental, receptive space. The neurons in our locus coeruleus may never be replaced, but the effects of this loss can be ameliorated as our capacity for co-organized neuroplasticity allows us to weave supportive circuitry around the injured parts" (Badenoch, 2018, p. 108).

RIGHT BRAIN ORIENTATION OF THE CLINICIAN AND CLIENT, TRAUMA WORK, AND EXPERIENTIAL UNITY THEORY AND MODEL

There is now consensus that deficits in right brain relational processes and resulting affect dysregulation underlie all psychological and psychiatric disorders. All models of therapeutic intervention across a span of psychopathologies share a common goal of attempting to improve emotional self-regulatory processes. (Schore, 2014, p. 390)

Allan Schore outlines the essential role the right brain plays in the unconscious processing of emotional stimuli, and the importance of therapy in engaging one unconscious mind with another unconscious mind. He states:

In accord with a relational model of psychotherapy, right brain processes that are reciprocally activated on both sides of the therapeutic alliance lie at the core of the psychotherapeutic change process. These implicit clinical dialogues convey much more essential organismic information than left-brain explicit, verbal information. Rather, right brain interactions "beneath the words" non-verbally communicate essential nonconscious bodily-based affective relational information about the inner world of the patient (and therapist). (Schore, 2014, p. 390)

Pat Ogden (2009), founder of Sensorimotor psychotherapy, concurs with a right brain bias in therapy. She reiterates the right hemisphere as the source of non-verbal communication of emotion. She also emphasizes the need for the list-making left hemisphere to take a hiatus in therapy to allow for emotional engaging in the "co-construction" of the therapeutic process. She purports that if rational thinking is sequestered, the languaging part of the brain can connect with the other part and assist in the integration of the hemispheres (Ogden, 2009).

Linda Graham, marriage and family therapist, purports:

We're emphasizing right brain to right brain here because it's an essential counter-balance to the dominance of the left brain in most of our dealings with clients, and because, for healing early attachment and affect regulation patterns, since those patterns are one hundred percent implicit (outside of awareness) it's the only thing that works. (Graham, 2004)

In Experiential Unity model, metaphor and drawings are used to engage both the clinician's and client's right brain to help bypass the conscious mind. Additionally Experiential Unity model utilizes mindfulness, visualization, and other somatically oriented techniques to connect with "sensations as a way of knowing" and exploring symptoms of nervous system dysregulation that have surfaced in the body. Over decades a great deal of research has been done on "brain dominance" theory and it has assessed the different functions, processes, problems, and information processed by the different hemispheres of the brain. A summation of this research below elucidates the importance of right brain engagement for emotional processing and therapeutic alliance. Below are descriptors of the left and right hemispheres of the brain:

Left Hemisphere
- Uses logic/reason
- Thinks in words
- Deals in parts/specifics
- Will analyze/break apart
- Thinks sequentially
- Identifies with the individual
- Is ordered/controlled

Right Hemisphere
- Uses emotions/intuition
- Thinks in pictures
- Deals in wholes/relationship
- Will synthesize/put together
- Thinks simultaneously
- Identifies with the group
- Is spontaneous/free

Experiential Unity model elicits the theme for a drawing or metaphor from the "here and now" processes of the group, or individual, in a therapy session. The co-construction of the image activates the right brain processes in both the clinician and client. According to Ian McGilchrist,

metaphor embodies thought and places it in a living context. These three areas of difference between the hemispheres—metaphor, context, and the body—are all interpenetrated one with another. Once again it is the right hemisphere, in its concern for the immediacy of experience, that is more densely interconnected with and involved in the body, the ground of that experience. Where the right hemisphere can see that metaphor is the only way to preserve the link between language and the work it refers to. (McGilchrist, 2018, p. 118)

The development of the image reflects the uniqueness of the group or individual process at that time. It also maintains the right-to-right brain orientation during the therapeutic engagement and pays attention to the presenting symptoms of nervous system dysregulation and activation of feelings. The image or metaphor is also focused on representing the embodied emotion that has resulted from a traumatic experience. For example, an individual or a group may reflect on a theme of "feeling out of control and lost." A visual representation of their current emotional state could be; for instance, floating down a turbulent river in a small vessel or boat and being tossed about by the currents. The vessel takes one direction and then another without any clear path forward. For Experiential Unity model the first task, if the client or group affirm that they relate to the image, is to draw it. In an individual counseling session utilizing the Experiential Unity model, the clinician or the client draws the image depending on client interest and ability. In a group session, one of the co-facilitators of the group constructs the drawing. Then, continuing with the above metaphor a heart is drawn on the figure in the boat. The session would initially focus on what emotion is coming up when you find yourself in a vessel on a turbulent river feeling lost and "out of control." Significant time is used to flesh out as many feelings as possible; for instance, disempowered, helpless, hopeless, confused, disoriented, destabilized, directionless, vulnerable, fear, uncertain, frustration, and lonely. In both group and individual sessions, clients are often asked at this point if any emotions listed in the drawing were experienced repeatedly in childhood. An asterisk is put next to those feelings to highlight the longevity of implicit memory held in the person's body and feelings and sensations that are often reflective of past trauma.

Once the traumatic embodied emotion is elucidated and sensations acknowledged, the right-to-right brain focus continues with expanding the drawing to fully reflect the complexity of the clients' present experience. For instance, it may be helpful to ask the individual or group "What obstacles do you see ahead of you in the river?" as a way of unpacking future fears and concerns. In the drawing it may also be key to illuminate past traumatic events, such as representing the past distress by large rocks in the river that the client has endured as a way of emphasizing resilience and fortitude in their struggle. To continue with the boat metaphor, or drawing, and maintain a right brain orientation, imagine whirlpools under the boat that are dragging the individual or the group down into a vortex. Naming what is contributing to the "dragged down" feeling can be helpful as clients are then alerted to unhelpful forces that are negatively impacting their situation. It could be personal actions or inactions; for instance, drinking more alcohol to cope or being passive physically. Each image in the Experiential Unity model is intent on developing a full understanding of the extent of the struggle felt by the client in an individual session or clients in a group setting. Once both the clinician and client have a fully fleshed-out version regarding the present situation represented by the boat in a turbulent river, the drawing then focuses on a path forward. The path forward is a counter-experience to the initial one of feeling "out of control" and "lost." This could be represented in a variety of ways; for instance, perhaps there is a bird up head that can see a path forward with a detached perspective. Imagining any way out is often extremely challenging when experiencing trauma. Or the person in the boat could pull out binoculars and see a less turbulent portion of the river up ahead. Utilizing imagination and creativity (right brain processes) of both the client and clinician help create a way out of the present felt experience of "being out of control" and "lost." This is a critical piece in trauma work—the traumatic experience in the form of sensation, urges, and feelings are felt at such intensity and can often trigger a traumatic freeze, fight/flight, or dissociative response. Often managing the moment and moving forward appear impossible and consequently keep the client stuck. This process of the path forward would then be fully explored using right brain processes that draw on intuition, expresses itself in pictures, exercises spontaneity and the art of synthesizing to name a few. I have noted how relieved clients are when they have both understood the complexity of their struggle and mapped out a path forward. Also, clients have remarked that the drawing is a highly accurate representation of their "felt" experience; the fact that it was co-created by the clinician and individual client or clinician and group members offers an experience of "being understood by an empathic other"—a critical piece of trauma work. As stated by Bonnie Badenoch (2018) the essence of trauma isn't events, but the aloneness within them. "Who we perceive as being with us before, during, and after an event is central to our ability to integrate the trauma throughout our embodied and relational brains" (Badenoch, 2018, p. 25).

In summary, with the visual mapping process clients relive the event through the drawing in a detached way; the detachment assists them in staying within their ability to cope with the nervous system dysregulation related to past traumatic experiences. With both clinician and client engaging in right brain processes, the client experiences being with an attuned other. This gives the client an opportunity to explore secure attachment with the therapist in a mutual ventral state and potentially creates a correctional experience.

In contrast to right brain processes, the left brain attention to specifics, particularly the details of the traumatic event, and the analysis of "what happened" can be triggering. Using logic and reason to understand the trauma in a sequential manner can contribute to the client reliving the traumatic sensations and feelings. It is key to note that implicit memory is often not recollected in a sequential manner but rather as shards of memory given the amygdala's role in storing implicit memory. This process of going over the details of the traumatic experience (a common experience in mental health assessment interviews and some counseling sessions) has the potential to move the client outside their "Window of Tolerance." The term "Window of Tolerance" was coined by Dr. Dan Siegel in 1999 and is now commonly used to understand and describe normal brain/body reactions, especially following an adversity. The process of recollection of the traumatic event can often trigger an autonomic nervous system response. Babette Rothschild developed a six-category chart outlining a range of responses that the client could experience. They include parasympathetic-lethargic I (PNS I), parasympathetic-calm II (PNS II), sympathetic active / alert I (SNS I), fight / flight sympathetic II (SNS II), hyper freeze sympathetic III (SNS III) and hypo freeze parasympathetic III (PNS III) and dorsal vagus collapse. Rothschild highlights the need for particular attention to be paid to

the low energy of someone who is very sad, aggrieved, or depressed, and the state of hypo arousal collapse that may occur during or in the immediate aftermath of a life-threatening event, or more rarely, in one suffering from severe PTSD. The first one, PNS I, is the result of a deficit of energy. PNS III hypoarousal is, on the other hand, the result of overwhelming arousal which causes a nervous system shutdown that leads to collapse. PNS III hypoarousal is the result of going over the top. Thinking in those terms will help you to distinguish that as a state of excessive overwhelm rather than an absence of vigor. (Rothschild, 2021, p. 48)

Tracking the clients' reactions to any material discussed in the session is critical; this moment-by-moment observation is a key piece regarding the client staying within the Window of Tolerance. If therapeutic engagement (without careful monitoring) repeatedly triggers the client, this can reinforce a sense of hopelessness and helplessness to deal with past traumatic events. Pat Ogden reiterates this point:

Clients suffering from unresolved trauma nearly always report unregulated body experience; an uncontrollable cascade of strong emotions and physical sensations, triggered by reminders of the trauma, replays endlessly in the body. This chronic physiological arousal often is at the root of the recurring post traumatic symptoms for which the client seeks therapy. (Ogden, Minton, & Pain, 2006, p. 28)

Bottom-Up Processing, Trauma-Focused Work, and Experiential Unity Theory and Model

Traditional talk-based psychotherapy, and most cognitively oriented trauma-based therapies, are viewed as taking a top-down approach to treatment. Most often this involves efforts to resolve trauma symptoms by working with the *dorsolateral prefrontal cortex*, the area of the brain most responsible for logic and reason. (Spinazzola & Wilson, n.d.)

A top-down processing approach assumes that the prefrontal cortex, with its capacity for reasoning, will be able to have a marked influence on the limbic system. The limbic system receives information from many body parts, including the heart, vagus nerve, gut/digestive system, and skin, and because of the hypothalamus's functions, the limbic system is directly in control of one's stress response. However, as Bessel Van de Kolk explains in a NICABM video that this top-down approach focused on recruiting the cognitive capacities of the mind is not helpful for working through trauma, "most of the therapies I am advocating here is limbic system therapy, trauma therapy is not about understanding or figuring things out, because that is really not where the trauma sits, trauma sits in automatic reactions, and your dispositions and how you interpret the world. In order to rewire the automatic perceptions, you need to have deep experiences that for your survival brain contradicts how you are now disposed to think" (NICABM, n.d.) Additionally, talking about a traumatic event and cognitively trying to process it can activate the dorsal vagal pathway which reacts to cues of extreme danger. Therefore, through conversation the body can relive the event as if it is happening right now. If danger is perceived the dorsal vagal "takes us out of connection, out of awareness, and into a protective state of collapse. When we feel frozen, numb or 'not here,' the dorsal vagal has taken control" (Dana, 2018, p. 9).

Bottom-up processing on the other hand refers to processing sensory information as it is being experienced in the moment in a relationally attuned therapeutic milieu. Body-based and somatic therapeutic interventions are focused primarily on connecting with "sensations as a way of knowing" and tracking nervous system dysregulation.

Experiential Unity model uses bottom-up processing as a way to engaging the client's somatic experience. Through their sensory experience the full impact of trauma and how it is impacting their everyday coping can be slowly pieced together. However, some clients experience a high degree of activation with somatic engagement, in those situations images or metaphors can be drawn that reflect the client's current situation, filling in the details of the drawing with a bottom-up processing technique.

In an individual client session with Experiential Unity model, a bottom-up process explores the client's felt sense of what is happening "in the moment" in their body. First, safety is established and what helps the client calm their body is ascertained. Then, through mindfulness and breathwork, and exploring sensation in the body, implicit memory contained in the body is engaged and helps in guiding the session. For example, a client after breathwork may feel tension in their shoulders; the session stays focused on the sensation and explores the shoulder area to see if other nuances of sensation are evident, and any emotions can be felt. The emotion identified may be, for instance, helplessness; the session then focuses on what the helplessness is about. The emotion identified may relate to their present distressing situation or not. It may have been triggered by their present issues. From a trauma-informed perspective, it is critical to integrate emotions that have surfaced, as it is a key piece in supporting the change process; another critical piece is for the practitioner to stay relationally present. Many individual clients I see start out the session with strong ideas about what they feel needs to be the focus of the session that day. I respond by saying let's engage your body through breathwork and see if the body has a different idea of what is critical to explore today. Most often the body has a unique focus, and the client is alerted time and time again that what they think is really going on may or may not be relevant to their healing.

Experiential Unity model continues with a bottom-up process through a mutual development of a visual image or metaphor which reflects the identified embodied emotion. For example, helplessness in the shoulders could be depicted by the client standing on quicksand, and no matter what they do they feel helpless to help themselves. The image is explored by eliciting information from the client to gain a deeper understanding of how "helplessness" is experienced by this client.

A similar process is used in group work. Experiential Unity model with a group starts with mindfulness or another calming technique and a group round of identifying feelings. The theme of the group is then elicited from the feeling rounds and the overall "check in" for the week. The bottom-up processing continues with the client's sensory information and key aspects of their trauma history included in the drawing or metaphor. The clinician then continues to ask questions that help to develop a fuller understanding of what the client in an individual session, or group members in a group, is experiencing at a deeper level. It is the client's sensory experience including tension and sensation felt in their body, urges, visuals, ideas, insights, feelings, reactions, observations, internal processes, and beliefs about self and self-awareness that is captured in the image which aligns with a bottom-up process. Barriers to change, and reflecting on helpful paths out of the predicament, are also key pieces to include in the image. This bottom-up processing engagement has demonstrated numerous advantages that have been observed over time.

- Clients have mentioned that the images are powerful because they reflect their current predicament on a somatic level and also build on their knowledge of their history of trauma.
- Clients have stated that they feel understood at a deep level.
- The images are filled in with client's thoughts, feelings, sensations, somatic experiences, and their ideas as some examples, so their role in their healing is very active and engaged throughout. This assists with a feeling of empowerment and reduces dependency on the clinician that can occur over time.
- The images and metaphors are take-home tools so the therapeutic engagement can continue post-session. Clients are encouraged to keep adding to the drawing, so the visual images become a support system between sessions.
- Clients have stated they are reminders of where they want to go in terms of self-growth and remind them of the positive changes they have already made.
- The images can assist clients in identifying and moving through barriers to change. In Experiential Unity model a great deal of attention is paid to obstacles to progress. From a trauma informed perspective; for instance, these could be core beliefs formed from an experience of trauma. For example, a core belief that comes up repeatedly is "not good enough." Core beliefs and patterns of behavior are often included in the drawings to give a more complex and nuanced understanding of the change process.
- The images unpack emotions that are felt in the body and sensation often outside of awareness, educating the client about the impact of embodied emotion and sensations as a way of knowing.
- Clients can explore themes that keep re-surfacing in their lives through the drawings.
- Visual images or metaphors assist clients in getting a "bird's-eye view" to their predicament often very challenging when immersed in a cycle of trauma.
- The images help clients bypass their intellect; it is particularly helpful to clients who are prone to analysis.
- The clients teach themselves—it is their process made visible.

As Bessel van der Kolk, author of the bestselling book *The Body Keeps the Score* and one of the leaders in establishing the scientific foundations of body-based therapy, puts it, the imprint of the trauma doesn't sit in the verbal understanding of the brain but lies in much deeper regions—amygdala, hippocampus, hypothalamus, brain stem—which are only marginally affected by thinking and cognition. People process their trauma from the bottom up—body to mind—not top down. For therapy to be effective, we need to do things that change the way people regulate these core functions, which doesn't usually occur through words and language alone. Arguably, over the past two decades, the advent of bottom-up psychotherapy—fueled by a range of clinical, scientific, and cultural developments—has been the most influential movement in the field of psychotherapy to date. (Dockett, 2013)

A bottom-up processing technique is also critical to acknowledge the impact of intergenerational trauma or historical trauma. Through somatic engagement implicit memory may reveal past trauma related to experiences of past generations. Resmaa Menakem in his book *My Grandmother's Hands* states:

We are only beginning to understand how these processes work, and there are a lot of details we don't know yet. Having said that this is what we know so far:

- A fetus growing inside the womb of a traumatized mother may inherit some of that trauma in its DNA expression. This results in the repeated release of stress hormones, which may affect the nervous system of the developing fetus.
- A man with unhealed trauma in his body may produce sperm with altered DNA expression. These in turn may inhibit the healthy functioning of cells in his children.
- Trauma can alter the DNA expression of a child or grandchild's brain, causing a wide range of health and mental health issues, including memory loss, chronic anxiety, muscle weakness and depression.
- Some of these effects seem particularly prevalent among African Americans, Jews, and American Indians, three groups who have all experienced an enormous amount of historical trauma. (Menakem, 2017, p. 40)

Experiential Unity model is aligned with bottom-up processes, but it is also possible to incorporate some top-down processes in the visuals. For instance, in the processing of the image or metaphor a CBT orientation can help unpack how the present experience is impacting thoughts, feelings, and behaviors. A cognitive approach could also include a bird's-eye view analysis of thinking patterns and developing awareness. Decision making, another top-down process, can also be advantageous in working with a client with an Experiential Unity model focus. Decision making can be included in the image or metaphor as focusing on a way out of distress. For instance, if the client is experiencing life in "quicksand" enquiring with the client what may help to get them to firmer ground.

The use of metaphor or a visual image in Experiential Unity model is from a neuroscience perspective helpful for accessing the medial prefrontal cortex. According to Dr. Joseph Spinazzola, in an article on the Complex trauma.o rg website, the medial prefrontal cortex is the "brains secret side door." The article goes on to explore the role of

> participation in expressive-arts based interventions such as theater, storytelling, and the visual arts, also seem to reach the medial prefrontal cortex through their drawing upon powerful cultural healing rituals and symbolism deeply rooted in the human experience which resonates with the human mind and spirit in a way transcending or at least circumventing the limits of logical thinking. These side door interventions appear to possess the potential to help guide complexly traumatized individuals towards a more integrated awareness and processing of unresolved trauma symptoms and reactions, helping to reset the thinking and feelings centers of the brain and to release the stranglehold of complex trauma on the body. (Spinazzola, & Wilson, n.d.)

In conclusion, Experiential Unity model, which includes a bottom-up processing approach, in relation to connecting with somatic memory and sensations and through accessing the medial prefrontal cortex via images, assists the client in processing traumatic material.

FOCUS ON IMPLICIT (EMBODIED) MEMORY FOR TRAUMA-FOCUSED WORK AND EXPERIENTIAL UNITY THEORY AND MODEL

Implicit memory is defined as unconscious or automatic memory. It contains the felt sense of an experience and the memories are held as "urges of feeling, behavioural impulses, bodily sensations, and perceptions that, when reawakened, color everything because implicit memories have the felt sense of happening now no matter how long ago, they may have been encoded" (Badenoch, 2018, p. xvii). Bonnie Badenoch goes on to say as human beings we encode 11 million bits of sensory information per second on an implicit level, while only encoding 6 to 50 bits on a conscious, explicit level, suggesting that implicit memories are being stored at a much greater rate than explicit memories; these often-unconscious implicit memories influence our everyday life dramatically, shaping our perceptions and thoughts and overall feeling state (Badenoch, 2018, p. xvii). An understanding of the impact of implicit memory is critical in terms of trauma-informed practice. It plays a key role in understanding the "reliving of trauma and the activation of trauma." Implicit memory or embodied memory can be triggered by shards of sensory experience; for instance, an abusive parent may be associated with the smell of smoke and so the smell of smoke, often below conscious awareness, may trigger a wide range of feelings and flood the body with sensation as if the event was happening right now. This is termed by Badenoch as implicit memory being "the eternally present past" (Badenoch, 2018, p. 167). When the same implicit memories are relived over and over again, they are termed "embodied anticipations" and in essence they form expectations of how our lives will unfold. These embodied anticipations impact our perceptions of our lives as a whole, influencing sensation in our bodies, beliefs, thoughts, actions, and ideas. Patterns of relating, and patterns of behavior, can provide clues as to the effect of "embodied memory and anticipations." For example, if a client is in a perpetual cycle of self-sabotage there may be embodied memory around inadequacy and not feeling good enough, hence the unconscious self-sabotage keeps re-occurring.

In working with embodied emotion and body memory it is key to understand the differing types of body memory:

- Habitual or procedural body memory: This memory is utilized for familiar activities like driving a car; it "refers to the habitualisation of the sensorimotor capacities of the lived-body" (Koch, Caldwell, & Fuchs, 2013, p. 83).
- Situational or body memory: "Memory of spatial familiarity (for interior and exterior spaces) and atmospheric perception. Situational memory extends into the spatio-temporal situation in which we bodily participate. As such, it entails the involuntary emergence of memory images and impressions that are related to the atmosphere of certain (mostly affectively charged) lived situations" (Koch, Caldwell, & Fuchs, 2013, p. 83). This assists us in our connection with certain situations and detachment from others.
- Inter-corporeal body memory: This memory is formed early on in life, and it forms an implicit template for our body reactions to engaging with others. These body memories assist in developing an implicit knowing of how to deal with others and form relationships.
- Incorporative body memory: This body memory relates to the adoption of certain mannerisms pertaining to identity. It can relate to gender roles and physical expressions related to personality. It is most often influenced by familial and societal expectations of self.
- Pain memory: This is the internalization of pain and a remembering that guides the present moment.

- Traumatic memory: Traumatic memories are past experiences of intense suffering that are still impacting the present. At times they are not recollected and can manifest in a variety of psychosomatic illnesses as a way of expressing the past distress. "In trauma, the feeling of 'at-homeness' is often lost and needs to be regained" (Koch, Caldwell, & Fuchs, 2013, p. 83).

Many models of therapy emphasize choice, detaching from negative thinking patterns, assessment and analysis to resist self-defeating tendencies, and exploration of alternative thoughts. For example, CBT uses knowledge of thinking patterns like "all or nothing thinking" or "catastrophizing" to assist the client in distancing from the thinking pattern that is having an impact by disputing it. A common tool applied to challenging situations using the CBT model is the "thought record." The thought record uses a variety of categories—for instance, situation, feelings, unhelpful thoughts, facts that support unhelpful thoughts and then facts that provide evidence against the unhelpful thought. The last two categories encourage alternative, more balanced perspectives and outcome. I have witnessed some clients feel empowered by this process; the thought record helped them distance from the depth of distress they were experiencing and develop perspective. Alternatively, I have also observed clients in a coping with depression group criticize themselves because they are still consumed by the negative thinking pattern. Clients have articulated that "there must be something wrong with me" or "I am a particularly hopeless case as I am not able to control my thoughts, manage my emotions and feel better." The role of implicit memory is a key piece in understanding how much change is possible without addressing implicit or embodied emotion. As Linda Graham states in *Bouncing Back*:

> It's humbling to realize the power of our implicit memories: anything we learn or come to believe later in life, about ourselves, about others, or about how the world works, can be overridden or hijacked by our earliest learning. And it often is. We can experience that response from implicit memory with such force and vividness that we have no sense whatsoever that we're experiencing an emotional flashback to our earliest ways of coping rather than something that is happening now. (Graham, 2013, p. 39)

Implicit memories have no time stamp, therefore they can intrude at any time, for instance it may be a memory related to fear. This memory will now influence the person that their dreaded fear is true and will most likely be long lasting.

Experiential Unity theory and model, in both Individual and Group therapy formats, incorporates implicit memory by utilizing mindfulness, breathwork, sensations as a way of knowing, and movement as a way of accessing embodied, implicit memory. This is critical from an integrative perspective as the embodied emotion in the unconscious is responsible for influencing how the client feels at this moment in time, has the potential to trigger unhelpful thinking patterns, and can also be the instigator of fixed and challenging patterns of behavior that are very difficult to undermine. For instance, Linda Graham states "As human beings we pride ourselves, and rightfully so, on the phenomenal capacities of our higher, 'thinking' brain to learn from past experiences, sort through complex issues, and resolve current problems. We recall previous coping strategies that were processed consciously and stored in explicit memory; we intentionally reflect on our opinions and deliberately choose the best strategy for current circumstances" (Graham, 2004). "However," Graham continues, "we may be giving too much credit to the higher brain for these responses. Neuroscientists have discovered that about eighty percent of the neural instructions for behaviour are recorded in implicit memory, outside our conscious awareness" (Graham, 2013, p. 36).

When clients are able to connect with "sensation as a way of knowing" to access embodied emotion, or implicit memory, name it, sense its historical meaning if they can, and use a technique to integrate and metabolize experiences that have not been processed, there is noticeable relief in nervous system regulation. This is a key piece in Experiential Unity model and may contribute to the amount of change clients are able to achieve over a short period of time. Other mind/body modalities like somatic experiencing (Levine, 2015) align with the same principle re-attuning to sensation, titrating with a small dose of survival-based arousal, and resourcing with attuned social engagement and self-regulation to develop a corrective experience. In Experiential Unity model clients in both formats are invited to engage in a technique they find calming and grounding and that helps them to access implicit memory while attuning to social engagement with the clinician. This technique assists them in experiencing sensation, urges, tension, or emotion in their body at that time and therefore helps to engage implicit memory. Clients are asked to name a feeling if they can sense one and then explore what the feeling may relate to. A variety of techniques are then utilized to explore the full meaning of the implicit memory and understand it with regard to the client and their history, and expand awareness on its impact. The implicit memory can assist the client in illuminating a present pattern of behavior that has been challenging to transcend and help the client in exploring barriers to progress. Implicit memory and resourcing are active throughout the session by noting the client's nervous system dysregulation and using titrating and pendulating.

ONGOING TRACKING OF AROUSAL FOR TRAUMA-BASED WORK AND EXPERIENTIAL UNITY THEORY AND MODEL

A further key tenet of Trauma-informed Practice, which is incorporated into Experiential Unity theory and model, is the Window of Tolerance and the ongoing tracking of hyper- or hypoarousal. The term "Window of Tolerance" was first coined by Dr. Dan Siegel in 1999 (clinical professor of psychiatry UCLA) to understand and describe normal brain/body reactions, particularly when there are adverse events. The term, which has gained popularity since, suggests that there is an optimum level of arousal whereby emotions and sensory and cognitive activation can be tolerated, and that coping strategies are effective in dealing with the activation. The client is able to stay connected with the parasympathetic nervous system allowing for the processing of memory and emotions related to traumatic events.

Bessel Van De Kolk in a NICABM video talks about keen observation on the client's body as soon as he meets the client in their first session. Once the client walks into his office, he assesses eye contact and breathing and whether the client is "able to live within their rib cages." He states clearly that "if the primitive part of the brain is all up tight there is no use to do psychotherapy" and so he can spend the entire session encouraging the client to breathe so as to assist the latter in moving into their window of tolerance (NICABM, n.d.).

Experiential unity theory and model maintains a focus regarding the window of tolerance from the start of the first session and keeps self-regulation, and co-regulation, as paramount throughout the subsequent sessions. For self-regulation a key piece of information in the first session is to assist the client in discovering what calms and soothes their body. For some it may be breathing, for others tapping or movement. It is critical from a trauma-informed practice perspective for therapists to offer a wide range of vagal toning/grounding/calming and soothing techniques so that clients can practice and assess the impact of the technique on their body. I have known several clients who find slow breathing activating but find tapping on acupuncture points or some Kundalini yoga exercises calming for them and bring them into their window of tolerance. My basic assumption is each client is different, and each body is different, and what may work well to calm a person's body one day may not work in the next session; hence the need for a wide range of techniques to assist the client in nervous system regulation.

In addition to techniques for grounding and calming it is also important to consider the concept of dual awareness. Babette Rothschild states, "Dual awareness in the sensory nervous system, that is, achieving a balance between perception of the exteroceptors and interoceptors – external and internal reality" (Rothschild, 2021, p. 62). It is common for individuals with a trauma history, for instance PTSD, to be excessively attuned to interoceptors for sensing safety, and this can lead to frequent dysregulation. In an opening therapy session, a key piece to incorporate is attention to the external cues in the environment; what do you see and hear, for example, as a way of balancing their experience and helping them maintain regulation.

Co-regulation is also a key piece in trauma-informed practice work. A definition for *co-regulation* or *mutual regulation* can be defined as the way in which one person's autonomic nervous system, sensitively interacts with another person's autonomic nervous system in a way that helps both achieve greater emotional and physical balance. "The brain learns and rewires itself best when it is calm and relaxed yet engaged and alert. Becoming present means 'showing up,' coming out of absentmindedness or distraction, out of denial or disassociation, into a mindful awareness of being here, now, in this body, and then gently sustaining this state of simply being as we rewire the brain's conditioned patterns of coping" (Graham, 2013, p. 90).

Experiential Unity theory and model incorporates co-regulation in both Individual and Group therapy formats. In an individual session when the client is using breathing, tapping, or movement to calm and stay within their window of tolerance the clinician is also engaging in the same activity. This aligns with coordinated mutual engagement and initiates a co-regulation process early on. From a Polyvagal theory perspective, co-regulation is identified as a biological imperative: "It is through reciprocal regulation of our autonomic states that we feel safe to move into connection and create trusting relationships" (Dana, 2018, p. 4). As both client and clinician are calming and grounding together, it also provides an opportunity for the client to connect internally to nuances of sensation or tension in their body and any emotions. It also gives the clinician time to experience any intuitive or sensory information about the client. For example, a client I had never met sat down in my office; when I had a moment to attune to her somatically and experience her body language, I sensed the client felt "overwhelmingly lost." I pictured the client on a river as a log bouncing around not knowing where her life was going. I shared the image with the client who proceeded to sob uncontrollably as she found the image profound in explaining fully what she was experiencing. Her reaction was powerful and the rest of the session was focused on "being lost and out of control" which helped the client address a root issue.

Experiential Unity theory and model group work also pays attention to co-regulation principles. Similarly, to the individual therapy process a group therapy session starts out with mindfulness and provides an opportunity for all group members and co-facilitators to co-regulate. The deep listening, responding, interacting, focusing, and experiencing aspects of group therapy provide the environment for co-regulation. From Stephen Porges and a Polyvagal perspective, "group therapy provides exercises to promote the neural circuits involved in co-regulation and emotional regulation" (American Group Psychotherapy Association, 2016).

EXPERIENTIAL PSYCHOTHERAPY, TRAUMA-FOCUSED WORK, AND EXPERIENTIAL UNITY THEORY AND MODEL

Experiential psychotherapy has its roots in client-centered, existential, and Gestalt approaches to psychotherapy. Historical principles of Experiential psychotherapy historically put an emphasis on a genuine, empathic relationship and the clients deepening of their experience. Experiential psychotherapy, having evolved from its original roots, now places more of an emphasis in its current form on the therapist's contribution to the change process. Gendlin (1981) built on this approach by incorporating the "felt sense" of the body with an experiential process to form a therapeutic style called Focusing-Oriented Psychotherapy. A key role in Experiential therapy is the ongoing need of balancing directiveness with responsiveness. There is continual questioning whether to go with the clients' process or intervene with a helpful directive. Experiential therapists err on the side of the client's experience given the clients are considered the experts and the final arbiters of their experience. In this form of psychotherapy, clients are encouraged to disagree with their therapists at any juncture. Experiential therapists foster this type of exchange by seeing their roles as merely facilitators. Their input is stated tentatively encouraging the client to affirm, or disagree, with the intervention, feedback, or ideas.

Currently, there is a wide range of experientially based therapies; some have a primary focus on the body, while others have a different focus for treatment. One premise of Experiential psychotherapy is that if one can re-experience or express repressed feelings from the past, then one has an opportunity to release the implicit memory or embodied emotion. I often say to clients "you have to feel it to heal it." The trapped implicit memory is often contributing to a client experiencing arousal and moving outside their window of tolerance into nervous system dysregulation; this can also contribute to the client re-enacting trauma-based beliefs related to the trapped emotion. For instance, if inadequacy is trapped in the body, the core belief system of "I am not good enough" maintains a hold and external accomplishments struggle to undermine the haunting voice of inadequacy. A case in point is a client I had worked with who had achieved many of his desired goals and won various achievements. As he went up on stage to accept a prestigious award, he recalls feeling overwhelming inadequate and was consumed with the idea of "not being good enough" despite winning the award.

Some examples of experientially based therapies and their critical role in trauma-based psychotherapy are Sensorimotor Psychotherapy, Somatic Experiencing, Whole body focusing, Accelerated Experiential Dynamic Psychotherapy (AEDP), Psychodrama, Expressive Arts therapy, Equine therapy, Affect Phobia therapy (APT), Intensive short-term dynamic Psychotherapy (ISTDP), Gestalt Therapy, Eye movement Desensitization Reprocessing (EMDR), Hakomi, and Dance therapy to name a few. Pat Ogden in *Trauma and the Body* (2006) talks about the need for the therapist to adopt an experimental attitude "a mind-set of openness and receptivity that is characterized by curiosity and playfulness rather than the effort of fear" when utilizing Sensiromotor psychotherapy (Ogden, 2006, p. 195).

An AEDP trainer, Hilary Jacob Hendel, summarizes the benefits of experiential work in four main points:

1. Experiential work actively cultivates a mindful, non-judgmental, compassionate stance that helps a person become aware of his/her inner experience which changes the brain for the better.
2. Experiential work helps people get in touch with their core emotions (sadness, fear, anger, joy, excitement, sexual excitement, and disgust) so patients come to know what they are feeling and learn how to use their emotions instead of being controlled by them.
3. Experiential work diminishes anxieties and other symptoms in predictable, reproducible ways, which is why it is considered healing-oriented as opposed to insight-oriented psychotherapy.
4. Experiential work teaches people to become their own therapist, giving them practical life skills to work with their emotions and the emotions of others in ways that are more constructive than they had before starting therapy. (Hendel, 2019)

For body-oriented psychotherapy, experiential work is critical because the clinician and the client are tracking body sensation in the present time "moment to moment." From Bill Bowens perspective, "A living body is always moving . . . that movement will express the psychological and the physical organizational patterns that this person is going through, including traumatic patterns" (Bowen, 2008, p. 1). A key piece of working experientially is paying attention in the moment not only to what the client is verbalizing but particular attention to gestures, micro movements, changes in posture, any changes in breathing during the session, and temperature changes. If the client suddenly flushes or exhibits a tic momentarily this is all information and helps with the critical tracking of what lies beneath the surface. For instance, a client I met for the first time said explicitly in the session that she didn't need to deal with any issues related to her father as she had worked through them. As she made this statement, I noted her eye twitched. I wondered at that moment if her statement was a defense and made a mental note to revisit her relationship with her father if she was open later. After I had interacted with the client for some time she opened up about her father and most of the future sessions were around this topic. According to Levine, "the triggers are the cues from our bodies themselves, that keep reactivating the sense of helplessness, of futility, of fear, of despair. And until there's a body experience that contradicts that experience, and gradually comes to replace that experience, people are locked in the trauma and unable to reengage into life" (Levine, 2008, p.1).

In Experiential Unity theory and model experiential work is utilized in a number of ways:

- From the first session experiential work is used to discover what techniques assist the client in calming, grounding, and connecting with their body to sensation, tension, urges, and surfacing feelings, and what helps to keep them within their window of tolerance. The techniques could include, for example, different ways of breathing, qigong, Kundalini yoga exercises, shaking, tapping, humming, meditation, or visualization.
- Experiential processes are utilized to gain access to implicit memory. This is an exploratory process and what works for a client to access feeling in one session may not work in another session. Clients differ markedly re their ease of access with some of them reporting feeling numb and that they are unable to access any feeling, sensation, or tension in their body at that moment. In that instance a drawing or metaphor is utilized to reflect their present struggle to facilitate accessing deeper material.
- Once a pervasive feeling in the body has been identified, for instance, helplessness in the stomach region, experiential processes are used to deepen an understanding of the emotion(s). Some clients may know what the emotion relates to while others may require more sensory exploration. One client I have worked with for a while is able to name a feeling she is experiencing in the present moment and then is instantly able to see an image right away, while others struggle to find the meaning related to the emotion. Some clients may feel the feeling and if it is so intense they move outside their window of tolerance in a variety of ways—so pendulating and titrating are key in an experiential process.
- In Experiential Unity model, once a feeling has been identified, and what it relates to in the past, an image is imagined that would fit the situation. For instance, the feeling may be inadequacy re caring for a sick relative, therefore a fitting image may be a relative in a deep hole and not being able to reach them with an outstretched arm. Given the work is experiential, one can only

ascertain a fitting image once the feeling and circumstances are known. Both client and clinician are working in the moment to find an image or metaphor that would reflect the intensity of the felt emotion. A variety of images may be proposed until the client resonates with a certain visual and agrees that it fits the present situation. Unpacking the image, and describing in detail the emotional impact of the circumstances, is another key piece of experiential work. To date, I rarely repeat the same image for different clients unless it is a group with fixed themes. At times there are some overlaps with some common issues like internal conflict or connection/disconnection visual tools, but overall each client is considered in a unique situation and therefore a unique image or metaphor is constructed in the moment.

- Experiential Unity model also requires experiential work around the process of choosing questions to deepen an understanding of the specific circumstance. The questions help to ascertain what other emotions are being triggered by this situation. What other complexities are impacting the issue? Are there any historical factors that are being triggered making the present situation harder to deal with? The above questions are examples of angles one may explore, but are not prescribed, as for the most part each situation and corresponding image is unique.

- Experiential Unity model also uses experiential processes throughout the session to keep tracking arousal. This helps to make moment-by-moment mutual decisions on whether the client can continue with the exploration process or whether they need to stop and re-resource themselves. The ongoing tracking of signs from the body, utilizing sensations as a way of knowing, and the clients' feeling state, as well as their capacity to explore the issue at a deeper level, are continually assessed by both client and clinician. Often clients can move outside their window of tolerance rapidly, so a range of resourcing techniques are established prior to the explanation so that these can be utilized in an urgent manner for calming and grounding. This is a markedly different process from primarily "talk therapy" models as a session can stop and restart innumerable times. "Many therapists question the appropriateness of interrupting clients in their narrative, or even during an out-of-control emotional outburst. Many psychotherapy educational programs encourage following clients in their process and never stopping them. However, at least when dealing with PTSD, it can actually be dangerous to allow or encourage destabilized or dysregulated clients to continue in such states when they are unable to stabilize and regulate on their own – a common reason many seek treatment in the first place" (Rothschild, 2021, p 64).

- A primary focus of Experiential Unity model and other integrative models is that unintegrated emotions are processed during the session and experiences that haven't been metabolized are processed to reduce nervous system dysregulation. This is key so the client is not overwhelmed and activated on leaving the session. The resourcing techniques solidified in the session can be utilized as a coping tool outside of therapeutic sessions.

Incorporation of a Variety of Integrative Techniques to Work Somatically for Trauma-Focused Work and Experiential Unity Theory and Model

Experiential Unity model uses a wide variety of mind/body techniques to assist the client in reducing symptoms of nervous system dysregulation related to trauma. Included below are some of the techniques utilized to access body sensation and memory, calm, ground and process unintegrated emotions. These coping techniques can be used throughout the session as a way of resourcing the client.

Breathing, Trauma Work, and Experiential Unity Model

> In several studies of trauma survivors including those who have survived sexual assault, incidences of fire and have been victims of crime, sleep disordered breathing (SDP) has at times been a consequence (Krakow et al., 2006, p. 433). Sleep disordered breathing encapsulates a wide range of conditions and includes loud snoring, sleep apnea, upper airway resistance syndrome, nightmares, insomnia as some examples. For some learning breathing techniques can be helpful and can assist in dealing with the symptoms of nervous system dysregulation related to trauma, including breathing issues. Psychological studies have shown that a breathing practice can be a helpful intervention to reduce levels of anxiety, stress, and depression in clients. (Ma et al., 2017, p. 874)

Others may find breathwork activating, and that sleep disordered breathing symptoms may increase, triggering them into dysregulation. Diaphragmatic breathing can be very challenging for those who live in a chronic state of activation. For example, other muscle groups take over for the diaphragm, such as intercostals, scalenes, sternocleidomastoids, pecs minor, and abs, and therefore the diaphragm at times become stiff and weakened, and this can be very challenging to use it for breathing. In *Yoga and the Quest for the True Self*, Stephen Cope describes some of what happens physiologically when the body's needs have been suppressed in the aftermath of trauma: "suppression of breath, abdominal inhibition and core strength diminished, and locked jaw—all of these are physiological indicators which end up inhibiting breathing" (Cope, 2018, pp. 225–226).

On the other hand, many clients I have worked with who have experienced trauma find breathing techniques helpful to connect to their inner landscape through sensation, emotion, and tension in the body and they are able to access their inner experience with some degree of ease. Experiential Unity model uses some of the techniques given below to assist in the process of connecting to embodied emotion and releasing it:

• Alternate nostril breathing (Nadi Shodhana)

   This particular technique is helpful in improving lung function, and lowering heart rate, blood pressure, and sympathetic stress. Origins of the technique are ascribed to Patanjali, a sage in ancient India and thought to be the author of a number of Sanskrit works, the most renowned are the Yoga Sutras in which pranayama (breathing techniques) is included.

   The technique is practiced by placing the right thumb gently over the right nostril and using the ring finger of the same hand for the left nostril. When the right nostril is closed the participant inhales through the left nostril at a slow pace, holding at the top of the breath, then breathing out through the right nostril using the ring finger to close off the left nostril. The process continues with breathing through the right nostril and out through the left, alternating fingers according to the nostril. Using the cycle for five to ten breaths is common. Each nostril activates the opposite hemisphere of the brain. The left nostril activates the right hemisphere and the right the left hemisphere. This assists in improving the connectivity between the hemispheres of the brain and balancing the mind, and calming overall.

• Somatic resourcing through breathing

   The autonomic nervous system helps to regulate the heart rate and the rate of breathing, and impacts the digestive processes without conscious awareness. According to Graham, "when we intentionally slow down and deepen our breathing, we are activating the parasympathetic branch of the nervous system in a positive way. We are conditioning our brain to calm down and return to our window of tolerance. Breathing slowly and deeply can deescalate a full-blown panic attack in a matter of minutes" (Graham, 2013, p. 216). Somatic resourcing through breathing can include a technique of a 4-7-8 breath, breathing in for four seconds through the nose, holding for the breath for seven seconds, and exhaling for eight seconds. It also can include box breathing 4-4-4 and as Graham suggests breathing in and out of the belly. All are ways of activating the parasympathetic nervous system and therefore help to reduce the impact of reliving trauma and the activation of the sympathetic nervous system.

• Bhramari Pranayama (bee breathing)

   Bhramari is a Sanskrit term which derives its name from Bee," as the exhalation sound produced in this pranayama resembles the humming sound of a bee. The pranayama is from an ancient yogic text Hatha Yoga

Pradipika (HYP) where it's described as one of eight classical breathing techniques.

The technique can be a powerful way to begin and end a therapy session as it has a wide range of benefits. Most clients I have worked with find it powerful for calming and helpful for connecting with implicit memory or sensation in the body. The Art of Living website recommends doing bee breathing through the following steps:

1. Sit up straight in a quiet, well-ventilated corner with your eyes closed. Keep a gentle smile on your face.
2. Keep your eyes closed for some time. Observe the sensations in the body and the quietness within.
3. Place your index fingers on your ears. There is a cartilage between your cheek and ear. Place your index fingers on the cartilage.
4. Take a deep breath in and as you breathe out, gently press the cartilage. You can keep the cartilage pressed or press it in and out with your fingers while making a loud humming sound like a bee.
5. You can also make a low-pitched sound, but it is a good idea to make a high-pitched one for better results.
6. Breathe in again and continue the same pattern 3–4 times.

The following precautions are advised by a Srisri yoga teacher at an Art of Living center:

- Ensure that you are not putting your finger inside the ear but on the cartilage.
- Don't press the cartilage too hard. Gently press and release with the finger.
- While making the humming sound, keep your mouth closed.
- You can also do Bhramari pranayama with your fingers in the Shanmukhi Mudra (closing 2 eyes, both ears and nostrils and mouth)
- Do not put pressure on your face.

Do not exceed the recommended repetitions of 3–4 times. (The Art of Living, n.d.)

Other benefits of this technique include calming those with hypertension, anxiety, and anger issues, and reducing blood pressure. Clients have reported that it clears the mind, which is helpful as often clients report that a busy mind can hinder deeper integrative therapeutic work. It also helps alleviate headaches and migraines.

Tapping for the Release of Embodied Emotion Related to Trauma and Experiential Unity Model

Tapping is another integrative technique utilized in the Experiential Unity model to assist in releasing embodied emotion or implicit memory. The origins of tapping date back to ancient Chinese medicine and acupuncture.

Acupuncture uses needles in the energy meridians, or energy pathways, to clear blockages in the system. It was developed initially to treat physical problems but later was adapted to focus on emotional concerns as well. Dr. George Goodheart (1975), a renowned chiropractor in the United States, experimented by applying simple manual pressure instead of the acupuncture needles and discovered similar results. Later in the 1970s an Australian psychiatrist Dr. John Diamond (1978) built on Goodheart's technique. Dr. Diamond experimented with stating affirmations, or positive self-statements, while tapping on the acupuncture points and used this methodology to treat emotional concerns. In the early 1980s Dr. Callahan (2001) took the techniques a step further to develop Thought-Field Therapy (TFT) combining kinesiology and the study of the meridian system of acupuncture. His focus was on clients with anxiety and phobias. He describes his techniques thus:

> When we think about an experience or thought associated with an emotional issue, we're tuning-in to a thought field. Perturbations are precisely encoded bits of information contained in our thought fields. And each deformity within a thought field is said to be connected to a particular issue (anxiety, depression, etc.)—and activated by thinking about it. (White, 2011)

Perturbations, according to Callahan, are at the foundation of negative emotions. He goes on to explain that each perturbation is linked to a particular point in the body and so tapping a specific sequence can assist in purging the issue from that source. The focus is to remove blockages in qi (energy) similarly to acupuncture. Gary Craig (1995), a Stanford engineer and student of Dr. Callahan, went on to create the Emotional Freedom Technique (EFT) in the mid-1990s. Craig adapted the tapping techniques for a wider application to also include an array of health problems such as migraines, facial neuralgia, back pain, and fibromyalgia.

Tapping or EFT has been used in several research studies. A narrative systematic review of six studies found that EFT may be an effective intervention for public speaking anxiety and test anxiety (Boath et al., 2017). In terms of test anxiety specifically, Benor et al. (2009) noted that EFT, compared to CBT, significantly lowered psychological distress with participants reporting positive qualitative effects and a willingness to use the therapy in other situations. Gaesser and Karan (2017) have also compared EFT to CBT and found using EFT resulted in significant reductions in adolescent anxiety in schools, especially compared to a wait-list control. Furthermore, Sezgin and Özcan (2009) reported that EFT may be more effective when compared against progressive muscular relaxation in reducing test anxiety and helping students score significantly higher grades post-intervention. However, the effects of EFT can be more subtle with Jain and Rubino (2012) suggesting that while there was a trend for "EFT to be more effective in reducing test anxiety by lowering distraction, compared to no treatment, other techniques such as diaphragmatic breathing appear more effective, by increasing calmness" (Boath et al., 2017). Qualitative research in the study included feedback from participants. Participants stated that they found EFT helpful for calming and reducing anxiety. Other participants found reduced physical sensations associated with stress.

Another research study focused on EFT to provide both help and support for social work students. A tapping intervention was utilized in the study to potentially benefit communication skills, preparation for practice placements, and the transition into a social work career. Qualitative research in the study included feedback from participants as well. Some participants stated they found EFT helpful for calming and reducing anxiety, while others found that it reduced physical sensations associated with stress. Protocols utilized for treatment with EFT require several specific steps.

- Tapping a part of the body to balance the energy in the body.
- A verbal statement that uses affirmations to reinforce the tapping intervention.
- Eye-roll (sometimes used in hypnotic treatment) can help stimulate communication between the left and right hemisphere of the brain.

Another study by Dr. Feinstein (2004) (PhD, clinical psychologist, executive director of the non-profit organization Energy Medicine Institute) and J. Andrade (2004) (MD, Medical Director of JA&A, Argentina) involved a group of 29,000 participants of which 5,000 were diagnosed with anxiety disorder. The participants were assigned randomly to an experimental EFT group and a control CBT/medication group. The study was conducted for over a period of five years and follow-ups included an in-person or phone interview at 1, 3, 6, and 12 months after the initial treatment.

Preliminary post-study results showed 76% of the experimental group members were judged as symptom free from anxiety compared to 51% of the individuals in the control group. At a one-year follow-up, the individuals who had received tapping treatments were less prone to relapse than those receiving CBT/medication. The results are remarkable but preliminary and not peer-reviewed. (Brattberg, 2008)

Experiential Unity model uses a variety of tapping techniques to assist in the release of embodied emotion. Jessica Ortner (2021), a renowned tapping specialist, has produced an online audio recording that includes six tracks that are designed to release overall stress. I have utilized this recording in a psychiatric group therapy program for a mindfulness and relaxation group, a crisis stabilization group, and a self-compassion group. Many clients have reported feeling calmer, more grounded, and more connected with their body. Some have reported a tingling feeling and a variety of other sensations in their bodies that they associate with relaxation. Over an eight-year period, there have also been clients that are uncomfortable with tapping, don't believe in it, and occasionally for some, it has contributed to more agitation or feelings of anxiety. Therefore, it is critical to point out at the onset that it is important to track "how your body feels" after any intervention to figure out "what works to help your body calm, ground and release."

A tapping technique that I have utilized that is helpful in releasing embodied emotion during the session, and for the clients to use if interested, between sessions includes the following steps:

1. Breathe, go inside, notice sensation and feel what you are feeling. Identify the "why" if possible.
2. Alternate tapping—with your thumb and first finger tap on the pads of the fingers about 4 times on the one hand, 4 times on the other hand, and continue the alternate tapping.
3. Keep up the tapping and say the mantra "Even though I feel ---------------- ---- (insert feeling) because of ------------------ (state why briefly) I deeply and completely accept myself."

Example: Even though I feel sad and helpless that my dog is in pain and the meds are not working I deeply and completely accept myself.
Say the mantra four or five times out loud if possible while tapping.

4. Now stop the tapping and breathe, sensing and intuiting if there is another feeling that has surfaced in your body.

Note: The mantra states "I deeply and completely accept myself." Some clients have reported they would like to believe the statement but that they struggle with self-acceptance. I often respond with the idea that stating it, whether you believe it or not, has positive effects on the brain. One study discovered that "saying affirmations increased activity in the medial prefrontal cortex and posterior cingulate. These areas of the brain are connected to self-related processing. Science shows that increased self-related processing can act as a kind of emotional buffer to painful, negative, or threatening information" (Hampton, 2019).

If clients are motivated to develop their own mantras for a specific issue, there are a wide range of examples on tapping websites under EFT.

• *Kundalini yoga poses to release embodied emotion related to trauma and Experiential Unity model*

The history of yoga is steeped in uncertainty given some of the first writings on yoga were transcribed on palm leaves. Pre-classical yoga can be traced to a civilization in Northern India called the Indus-Sarasvati civilization (Indus Valley Civilization) around 5,000 years ago. Yoga was developed over time by two cultural groups the Brahams and Rishis who documented beliefs and the practice of yoga in the Upanishads. Kundalini yoga was also recorded in the Upanishads between 1000 and 500 BCE and was initially considered a science of energy and spiritual philosophy, and later as physical practice. The science of Kundalini was kept hidden for thousands of years and was passed on in secret from a master to a chosen disciple who was considered worthy of the teachings. One disciple named Yogi Bhajan (born as Harbhajan Singh) after learning the teachings decided to travel to North America and consequently started to share the teachings. He had been hired for work by a university professor in Canada. He learned on arrival that the professor had died, and he also lost his luggage.

> There he was, September of 1968, in a strange country with no job, only $35, and the clothes on his back. . . . By introducing what he called the "Yoga of Awareness" to the West, *Yogi Bhajan* had broken an ancient tradition of secrecy. . . . He defied that tradition because he could see no logic in keeping these teachings from the thousands of young people out there who were abusing drugs in search of higher consciousness. His was an alternative to the drug culture. He knew that his technology would give seekers a real experience of God within, and also help them to heal their mental and emotional problems—as well as their physical bodies damaged by the use and abuse of drugs. Yogi Bhajan's legacy is under review given allegations that have surfaced.

Kundalini yoga in its present form consists of a blend of physical postures, breathing exercises (pranayama), meditation, and kriyas which are repeated body movements with an intent of facilitating the flow of energy in the body. It is practiced in many countries around the world and has also been used in a variety of research projects. Kundalini yoga as a treatment has been the subject of research by the Center for Addiction in Mental health in Toronto, Canada. Jindani and colleagues conducted an investigation to assess the impact of 8 weekly 90-minute sessions of Kundalini Yoga, including a 15 min of practice per day at home, would have on PTSD symptomology and increased well-being compared to a waitlist group for KY. The study was not conclusive due to some methodological limitations (Jindani & Khalsa, 2015).

In 1991, Shannahoff-Khalsa, the director of The Research Group for Mind-Body Dynamics at UCSD's BioCircuits Institute, and a member of the UCSD Center for Integrative Medicine and a pioneer in novel studies in the neuroscience, "published a chapter in a scientific book on stress that included Kundalini Yoga techniques for (1) treating anxiety; (2) treating fatigue; (3) stimulating the immune system for treating solid tumors; (4) expanding and integrating the mind; (5) developing a comprehensive, comparative, and intuitive mind; and (6) regenerating the central nervous system" (1991, p. 88). The Kriyas take the form of a list of instructions for a specific issue. The following example is one for treating fear:

TECHNIQUE 8: TECHNIQUE FOR MANAGING FEARS

This technique was first published in 1997, and again in 2003. Sit with a straight spine. Close the eyes. Place the left hand into the navel point, with the 4 fingertips and thumb grouped together, and press very lightly. Place the 4 fingers of the right hand (pointing left) over the third eye (on the forehead just above the root of the nose), as if assessing fever. Play the audio- tape of Chattra Chakra Varti for 3 minutes while consciously assessing any fears and relating to the mental experience of the fears. This technique is claimed to help manage acute states of fear and to help eliminate fearful images and negative emotions that have developed due to frightening events. The effect is that the negative emotions related to specific fears are replaced with positive emotions, thereby either acutely or over time creating a new and different mental association with the original stimulus. This technique is analogous to the practice of exposure and response prevention. However, it is not necessary to actually physically engage a threat or fearful situation. See the case study below for the use by a cancer patient in the latter stages of her disease and facing the fear of death (Shannahoff-Khalsa, 2005, p. 91).

Kundalini yoga is also employed in cancer care utilizing specific meditations for specific cancer symptoms. To date Kundalini yoga techniques have proven to be highly effective for clients with an obsessive-compulsive disorder diagnosis "and show nearly twice the efficacy rate when compared to conventional treatments for this otherwise 'recalcitrant disorder,' only future studies can determine how useful these techniques can be for cancer patients" (Shannahoff-Khalsa, 2005, p. 99).

Experiential Unity model has utilized Kundalini yoga for over an eight-year period in a psychiatric group therapy program to release tension, anxiety, anger, and symptoms related to trauma with a sequence of movements. The separate poses do not form one of Yogi Bhajan's kriya's, but are inspired by Kundalini yoga, and the permission to use them in this form has been granted by the Kundalini research Institute. Prior to wrap up of the group, a 10-minute sequence of Kundalini yoga and other exercises, for example, shaking, is offered to the clients in a crisis stabilization group, a mindfulness and relaxation group, and a self-compassion group. Music is played to accompany the experience, and clients who are comfortable and willing to take part in the exercise component are asked to turn their backs to the circle and copy the facilitator, so that each client has some degree of privacy. Each movement has a specific benefit and overall clients have reported feeling lighter, calmer, and more grounded, and also have felt their mood enhanced. Often clients state it was the most powerful part of the group given how they felt after the movement. Some clients have also reported tearfulness after the exercises and have understood it as their body's way of releasing emotion. The list of exercises includes the following:

Shaking: Start with five minutes of shaking—shaking any part of your body that you can, in any way that works for your body.

Shaking can take a variety of forms; for instance, TRE or Tension & Trauma Releasing Exercises created by Dr. David Berceli teaches a particular method of shaking. Peter Levine, a renowned trauma therapist who also guides clients in a form of shaking, wrote in his book called *Waking the Tiger* (1997) that animals don't get post-traumatic stress disorder because they shiver and shake their bodies once the danger has passed, thereby releasing the trauma from their bodies, and bringing their bodies back to homeostasis.

Continue with the following sequence role modeled by the facilitator:

Push-pull: With hands at chest level push outward from your heart with force pushing away what keeps you stuck. Then pull toward your heart what soothes you, what calms you, what uplifts and heals you?

Twisting: Arms bent at 90 degrees and elbows at shoulder level, twist left while breathing in through your nose and twist right and exhale through your nose. Then change breathing pattern inhale on right and exhale on left side. (Pose releases the build-up in the adrenals)

Pulling down quickly: With hands clasped directly over your head quickly pull your hands down to your stomach in a chopping wood motion keeping your back straight. (Release pressure from the heart)

Fighting the air: Breathe in and hold your breath—fight the air vigorously with your fists clenched for as long as you can while holding your breath. Breathe out when needed and repeat 3 times. (Release frustration and anger)

Airplane: Extend one arm up and hold the other arm extended down and move from side to side—breathing in on the one side and out on the other—change breathing pattern.

Moving arms backward and forward: With thumb tucked into the fist of each
hand move arms backward and then forward in large sweeping motion.
(Opening of the heart)

Alternate leg and arm lifts: Bring bent left arm on one side to right bent knee
on the opposite side together and change sides alternating opposite knees
with opposite arms. (Balance the two hemispheres of the brain)

Arms over back: Bend at your waist to a 90-degree angle with a flat back.
Raise your hands above your back and alternate opening and closing your
fists on each hand. (Helps to fortify nerves)

Breath of joy: Short breath in with your arms raised, short breath in with your
arms at the side, short breath in with your arms raised again and then bend
over completely and exhale through your mouth – repeat ten or more times.
(Helps to clear and reboot your body).

The Kundalini yoga exercises are also used for individual counseling sessions. Often, I use them separately; rarely have I gone through all the exercises in the above list in an individual counseling session. For instance, if a
client has worked through trauma and they appear heavy and weighed down
by the process I may introduce a breath of joy for clearing. I first demonstrate
it and then do it with the client to assist them with any awkwardness. I may
also use some of the other techniques; for instance, if anger surfaces, particularly if the client is uncomfortable with feeling anger, I may use punching the
air and holding one's breath. Again, I demonstrate it first and then take part
alongside the client. These are examples of attunement, attuning to the client,
their physical expressions and offering techniques if the client is open for
clearing with a kundalini yoga pose.

Mindfulness, Trauma-Based Work, and Experiential Unity Model

About 2,500 years ago, in texts such as *Satipaṭṭhāna* and *Anapanasati*, the
Buddha's teachings on the foundational principles of mindfulness were
transcribed. *Mindfulness* is considered a 'state of mind that appreciates the
flow of consciousness in the present moment with acceptance.' According to
Garland, Froeliger, and Howard, mindfulness practices involved two primary
components which are "focused attention" and "open monitoring." Focused
attention is the willful practice where attention is placed on an object as well
as acknowledging mental distractions while being in practice. The second
aspect, open monitoring, is "about noticing the present moment experience
without judgement" (Kathirasan, 2018, pp. 1–2).

Mindfulness and mindful meditation are powerful allies in trauma- and
somatic-based counseling. It helps the client track their reactions to experiences, and from a detached perspective become aware of choices and

opportunities to break unhelpful fixed patterns of behavior that may be part of an automatic dysregulated nervous system response. Mindfulness can also empower due to an observation of "what is happening" in the moment—one can then intervene when a symptom is at an early stage. In a men's anger management group, I co-facilitated for nine years, mindful awareness was utilized to intercept anger at an early stage, for instance, irritability. This early tracking assisted the men in the group to tackle their reactions by taking an early "time out." In the "time out" they could use mindfulness to get increased insight into what was triggering their anger, connect with any underlying feelings, and reflect on healthy choices re behavioral responses.

According to Linda Graham in her book *Bouncing Back*,

> research also shows mindfulness practices, even at this introductory level, increase the volume of the insula and improve its function of interoception—awareness of what is going on in the body. Better interoception strengthens our capacities for self-attunement, self-awareness, and self-empathy: it helps us track how physically comfortable, how emotionally nourished, and how relationally supported we feel. This in turn enhances the confidence in ourselves that increases resilience. (Graham, 2013, pp. 53–54)

Mindfulness is also key in connecting more deeply with implicit memory held in the body. According to Bessel Van De Kolk (2015), renowned psychiatrist, researcher, and teacher, a therapist's job is to assist clients feel and connect with their feelings, notice what is going on inside of themselves, and observe their sense of flow within their bodies in order to re-establish their sense of time. He also reinforces that some of the best therapy is primarily non-verbal.

Experiential Unity model uses a variety of mindfulness techniques to assist the client to connect with their bodies, to access embodied emotion, and to help build "sustained present moment awareness." In group work a range of mindfulness exercises are utilized; these can help the client observe how they are feeling in that moment in time. Clients also become increasingly aware of their thoughts and start the process of observing their thoughts more and develop some protection against getting caught up in a whirlpool of thinking. Some of the mindful practices utilized use breathwork to assist in the process. Clients slow down and become more aware of their inhale and exhale tracking it in the body along with sensations and feelings. In both Individual and Group counseling mindful practices and breathing techniques initiate the session for the client, and this helps the client get a deeper understanding of what emotions may be surfacing in their body which are critical for holistic counseling. Mindfulness and breathwork are also used periodically as urgent interventions in individual or group work if the client has moved outside their window of tolerance. In Experiential Unity model an individual session ends with some time for mindful reflection which gives the client a chance to gauge how their body has responded to the therapy session and how they are left feeling.

An example of a script may be as follows:

Find a comfortable place to sit and start to become aware of sitting on a chair or couch and how the cushion feels underneath your body. Closing your eyes or focusing your eyes on a point on the floor to help in the calming of your mind. Now bring attention to your breath becoming aware of your inhale and your exhale. Noticing how far your inhale can travel into your body, observing and noticing how your body is breathing. Where do you notice your breathing, do you feel it in your nostrils or are you aware of your chest rising and falling, noticing where you feel your body breathing. Your mind will wander from your breathing many times, let go of worrying that your mind has wandered, when you become aware come back to your breath and sensations in your body. When your mind wanders start to observe your thoughts as if they were leaves on a river, watch the leaves move down the river, seeing and observing your thoughts and notice that you are noticing your thoughts. Now put your hand on your heart as a reminder that you will be bringing kind attention to your breathing. Feel your hand rise and fall on your body, noticing sensations you are feeling in your body while you breathe with your hand on your heart. In the last few moments of this meditative state see if you can allow yourself to be right here, with nothing to do but breathe, and just nourish yourself in this moment accepting yourself just as you are. Pause . . . . When you are ready open your eyes and orient yourself slowly to the room around you, being aware of your body, releasing feelings and tension with your exhale, and bringing in all that you need with your inhale.

Visualization and Trauma-Based Work and Experiential Unity Model

According to neuroscience imagined experiences can be almost as powerful as an actual event for creating new neural pathways. Linda Graham writes "neuroscientists have discovered that the same neurons fire in our visual cortex when we imagine seeing a banana, as when we see one for real. When you use the power of your imagination to repeatedly visualize people supporting you, you are installing a pattern of coping in your neural circuitry that you can use as a refuge in times of difficulty or challenge" (Graham, 2013, p. 99). Dr. David Hamilton, a leading-edge scientist and author of a book, *How Your Mind Can Heal Your Body*, concurs. He talks about five reasons why people should visualize:

1. Empowerment—Dr. Hamilton talks about a potential shift with the tool of visualization, from an external locus of control to internal control,

using the imagination to take charge. With exercising self-power, a person starts to notice small incremental changes they are making toward a larger goal and they are likely more engaged in the process. He believes there is a shift in motivation when the person feels more empowered.

2. The brain doesn't distinguish real from imaginary—Dr. Hamilton writes. "Research shows that if one person does something and another person visualizes doing the thing, the same brain areas are activated in both of them. And if they keep doing the thing or imagining doing the thing, their brain regions undergo actual physical change (called neuroplasticity) to the same degree" (Hamilton, 2014). He reiterates harnessing the power of visualization to imagine health outcomes. He states a growing body of research that supports the role of visualization in improved results in health.

3. Dr. Hamilton also remarks that visualization can help with willpower and through the consistent use of the tool of visualization one is able to focus the mind more, and that increased focus has an impact on achievement of outcome.

4. Health benefits—Dr. Hamilton writes about the power of visualization to assist patients fight and recover from disease. Dr. Lazarus in an article *Can visualization techniques treat serious diseases* states "Thus, just as the mind's reactions to stress can impair immunity and promote illness, it is believed that certain mental processes, like specific images and visualization procedures, can stimulate the immune system to better fight disease" (Lazarus, 2016). He goes on to conclude, "While unequivocal and robust data supporting the efficacy of psychoneuroimmunology methods to fight serious diseases are still lacking, what is clear is that the process can have dramatic psychological benefits. The relaxation aspect of the method often produces greater physical and psychological comfort, and the idea that one's mind can be utilized as a potentially effective medical intervention gives one a sense of more personal control and greater optimism" (Lazarus, 2016).

5. Belief in visualization improves results—Dr. Hamilton mentions that when a patient takes a painkiller and the other a placebo, the results are strikingly similar. This is due to the person's brain producing a chemical reaction that aligns with the result the brain is expecting (Hamilton, 2014).

Experiential Unity model uses visualizations, as another integrative tool, to offer clients wanting to work through the impact of trauma and stabilize nervous system dysregulation. Visualizations are utilized in mindfulness exercises which can commence as both an individual counseling and group therapy session. The visualizations may be offered to assist the client in grounding and increasing their ability to "be present" in the session to access deeper material. It could include a wide range of imagined places—it may be situating themselves in a comfortable place in their home or taking themselves into the forest, a beach, or another place of escape where they tend to relax more fully. It may also involve imagining their feet going into thick, black soil and pushing them in deeper and deeper to ground more. Visualization can also assist the client to come into their body and rework a memory. Again, it is part of attunement, sensing, and intuiting what might assist the client at this moment to connect with their body and to access sensation as a way of knowing and embodied emotions.

Another way Experiential Unity model uses visualizations is as a tool to work through specific traumatic material in an individual therapy session. For instance, one client I worked with had a tough time with her family members, and often felt smothered by their neediness and their disregard for her boundaries. She imagined herself with wings over her heart whenever she was around them. Another client with a similar issue saw the family members in a separate carriage on a roller coaster, she was behind in her own carriage, giving her the feeling of separateness but still able to be around her family. Another client used a visualization to give back the projections she felt during childhood, for instance, "I am not enough" from her parents. Another example of utilizing visualization is a client seeing herself trudging up the mountain moving forward despite the struggle. She imagined her parents at the base of the mountain and used the visualization to consolidate the idea that her parents are not able to grow alongside her. Graham in *Bouncing Back* also gives examples of using visualizations in the healing process "Visualizing . . . can greatly enhance our ease and resilience as we face an unknown or frightening situation" (Graham, 2013, p. 99). This process helps with the ongoing rewiring of our neural circuitry that assists in coping in times of distress.

All the above integrative techniques are utilized in Experiential Unity model if the client is open and willing to experiment. The process is experiential and it may take trying several techniques to decide which are the most helpful. Some clients have said emphatically tapping doesn't work for them, but humming does. Their clarity around what works for their body is very helpful. Also, the body may change regarding what works, and we need to continually adapt to the body's changes. To date, I cannot recall a client who has not been interested in discovering what works for them and what assists them somatically in reducing the legacy of trauma in their bodies.

Chapter 3

Experiential Unity Model— Application to Individual and Group Therapy

Experiential Unity model was devised from clinical experience offering individual counseling in mental health programs, and working in various psychiatric group therapy programs for 30 years in Vancouver, Canada. As any dedicated clinician I was continually assessing what is working for clients, what assists in the change process, and what may create barriers to their progress. Over time in group therapy, I noted several overriding themes. One was the benefit that clients experienced by belonging to a group. Many would say after the first session that the piece that stood out the most was that they were not alone in their struggle. In an individualistically oriented society, I heard repeatedly from clients that they should be able to manage their problems on their own, that it was perceived by some as a sign of weakness to reach out for help. Another dominant theme in both individual counseling and group therapy was "I shouldn't feel the way that I do." I started to listen deeply to where clients had learned that only certain feelings were acceptable and other feelings they experienced; for instance, sadness or inadequacy, implied that they were failures or "not enough" in some way, or another overriding judgment about themselves. Many had categorized feelings into a positive or negative category, and the implication with the categorization is that the negative feelings should not be acknowledged and should be sequestered or suppressed in some way. Many had grown up in families that encouraged suppression of expressing emotions, and most clients related as well to living in a society where they had to keep up the appearances that they were successful. This meant pressure to only express "positive" feelings and being able to prove success with enough material acquisition. The consequence of these internalized beliefs was dramatic, clients reported repeatedly that if they felt any "negative feelings" they would instinctively get busy and distract from the feeling.

45

There were also other popular ways to numb; for instance, excessive work, drugs, alcohol, distracting with technology, and living a speed filled life and the consequent cerebral communication whereby they intellectualized their emotional experiences. Chapter four in the book describes these cultural traps to healing in a lot more depth, however here it is key to mention how lifestyle behaviors, considered the norm in this society, impact the client's ability to heal from traumatic experiences. Many clients attend individual counseling or group therapy with the intent of getting rid of depression, anxiety, low self-esteem, or other symptoms of distress. Numerous clients are not aware that there may be symptoms of past trauma—for instance, if hopelessness and despair are locked into the body due to the impact of living with a parent with addiction, the thought process triggered from the feelings may be "what's the point" and depression could likely be a consequence of the original trauma.

Also, it became apparent that clients who felt numb and couldn't name a feeling seemed to experience less relief from the therapeutic engagement offered in the program. This all made sense from a neurobiological perspective as Dr. Ruth Lanius (2017) describes the impact of trauma on the client's capacity to know what they feel and to remember relevant information. She describes the impact of trauma on the default mode network of the brain which comprises three areas. The posterior cingulate cortex is the area of the brain involved in sorting through what is relevant and what is not in their lives. This part of the brain is often impacted by trauma which is why a traumatized client may struggle with making wise decisions around discerning safety. Another part of the brain impacted by trauma is the dorsal medial prefrontal cortex, "that's an area of the brain that really helps us to know what we feel. It helps us to know our internal emotional life, so really to figure out what's going on emotionally inside. Again, when we think about our trauma clients, they have great difficulty from that, doing that. They're very much disconnected from their internal emotional life" (Lanius & Buczynski, n.d., p. 3). Lanius also describes the impact on the third region of the brain namely lateral parietal cortex whereby clients with a trauma history "often they don't know where their body starts and where their body ends. They're so disconnected from their own body and how their body relates to the environment" (Lanius & Buczynski, n.d., p. 3).

Experiential Unity model was devised to be able to work with clients where they are at, including clients who are numb, or others who had a low tolerance for acknowledging feelings and were intellectualizing their emotional experiences, and were impacted by trauma in a variety of ways. The drawings, images, or metaphors are tools to help clients build a tolerance to feelings, and to assist in bypassing their conscious mind and accessing deeper material. An image or visual, from a neuroscience perspective, offers a bridge between the prefrontal cortex and limbic system helping numb clients to be able to sense and access more feeling in their body. The visual images are flexible and can also incorporate aspects of Cognitive behavioural therapy, where applicable and intersperse some narrative therapy questions to enhance the image overall.

In devising a new model, I started to engage the clients differently. Clients' experiences in the "present moment" became a key focus, exploring somatically and utilizing calming strategies to gain access. For those clients that are unable to engage their body due to activation, the drawings are a way for them to develop a unique perspective regarding their present situation. Some clients find the body engagement in the session unnecessary and would rather start the session recalling all their current distress right away. To deal with this hesitancy I take the time to do an educational piece with the client, outlining the benefits of engaging the body in treatment, the reason for connecting with their world of sensation and feeling at the outset of the session, and the difference it can make if the session is aligned with the body, including micro-movements, gestures, breathing patterns, temperature changes, and body expressions. As Peter Levine states, "Therapists, by and large, are trained to work with the verbal communication. So, we kind of have to untrain ourselves a little bit, from just working with the words, to being interested in gestures, in the changes in posture, in changes in breathing, in changes in temperature which we see" (Bowen, 2008, p. 1).

Clients are also reminded if they talk in detail about distressing situations, they have experienced without engaging the body, they may leave the session feeling worse than when they started the session due to unresolved trauma being activated. Given the activation clients are alerted to a possibility of interruptions in order to stay within their window of tolerance.

Another observation that inspired the format of Experiential Unity model was the mismatch between the clients' present pre-occupations and the topic of therapy. In a group therapy program I worked in all material was pre-ordained for all the groups, for instance, a Coping with Depression group, Coping with Anxiety group, Self-compassion, Self-esteem, Crisis stabilization, Mindfulness and Relaxation group. Often the theme that emerged in the group from the check-in was unrelated to the pre-ordained topic. This is an ongoing strength of Experiential Unity model addressing what the clients are currently experiencing at that moment in either an individual or a group therapy format.

Another critical topic for therapeutic engagement that is included in the metaphor or image of Experiential Unity model is barriers to progress. From a trauma-informed perspective this is critical to highlight as clients need to develop a complex understanding of the power of belief systems and embodied emotion, and the extent that they influence their everyday choices. Building in barriers to progress into some of the images and metaphors, where relevant, assists the clients develop more self-compassion regarding impediments to their progress. They start to develop more self-awareness around what keeps tripping them up and can recognize patterns and work at circumventing them. For instance, learning that it is not their fault that they impulsively self-sabotage, or strive for perfectionism, even though they know consciously it sets them up for failure. Inserting the barriers to progress into the visual drawings when appropriate helps the client see the history of the pattern of behavior, and at times they can see that it is rooted back to childhood trauma in their family of origin. For instance, the drawing may be them feeling like a salmon swimming up the river, fighting one current after another. The currents can then be named as internalized barriers to progress. One current may be striving to please others at the expense of one's own needs. Another current could be neglect of self and an excessive fixation on others' needs. Whirlpools in the river could be included in the image to represent when the current takes hold and moves them into a powerful whirlpool of intense feelings, this is often where they are consumed by a vortex of self-criticism and self-loathing. Other barriers in the river could be large boulders which symbolize current stressors that they are facing in their life. Once all the barriers and anticipated hurdles ahead are represented, the focus of the drawing could be on ways to bypass the currents and whirlpools. This could be shown by the salmon moving to the side of the river where the currents aren't as strong. The client would then brainstorm what helps them in life keep to the side of the river and maintain steady progress. It could be strategies of self-care, developing awareness around personal patterns of behavior, and boundary setting with others using assertive statements. This is a critical piece in empowerment, a client's perception of reality and perceived barriers is built into the model in both individual and group therapy formats. Pat Ogden, founder of Sensorimotor psychotherapy explains "Much of what we see is colored and organized by what we expect to see. The cues towards which clients are compelled to orient, and which sustain their attention, are likely to be those that verify implicit beliefs held about self and the world. Susan had tendencies of orienting and attention that stemmed from beliefs formed through early relationship dynamics. She grew up with parents that were pre-occupied with their careers and each other, and she reported feeling unsupported and uncared for throughout her childhood. . . . The hypothesis or belief she formed was "no-one will ever be there for me, so I have to do it all myself." She did not notice offers of help from other people. Susan complained that her husband failed her in ways similar to those of her parents; however, her frustrated husband stated that he repeatedly extended support to Susan but that she consistently refused, or simply did not respond, so he had finally given up trying. Susan was clearly not orienting or attending to cues that would disprove her belief; instead, she focused on cues reminiscent of her past that verified her belief that no-one would support her" (Ogden, 2006,

p. 75). An example of attachment trauma compared to shock trauma that occurs after an unexpected traumatic event.

Another key aspect of Experiential Unity model that assists in the healing process is inclusion of the body in the drawings. Many clients have limited awareness about how trauma is held in the body and how it continues to influence their lives. Many drawings include what the body is experiencing at that moment; one drawing tracking the history of emotion (see visual 1.2) maps out the full impact of trauma on the body and the psyche. The drawing also assists the clients to get a deeper understanding that emotion is embodied, that it can be held in the body for decades, and that it has a profound impact on mood, ability to self-motivate, and a worldview that can be shaped by traumatic memory.

EXPERIENTIAL UNITY MODEL AND THE THERAPEUTIC USE OF IMAGERY, METAPHOR, AND VISUAL IMAGES IN CLIENT'S PROCESS

The use of images, metaphors, and visual images is a key component in the application of Experiential Unity model. As mentioned before the images and metaphors are a powerful way of engaging traumatic material and assist the client in processing and metabolizing past trauma. Use of imagery also aligns with the right-to-right brain orientation supported by neuroscience. As stated by Allan Schore (2014), American psychologist and researcher in the field of neuropsychology, "Neuroscience characterizes the role of the right brain in these nonverbal communications. At all stages of the life span, 'The neural substrates of the perception of voices, faces, gestures, smells and pheromones, as evidenced by modern neuroimaging techniques, are characterized by a general pattern of right- hemispheric functional asymmetry'" (Brancucci, Lucci, Mazzatenta, & Tommasi, 2009, p. 895). "More so than conscious left brain verbalizations, right brain-to-right brain visual–facial, auditory–prosodic, and tactile–gestural subliminal communications reveal the deeper aspects of the personality of the patient, as well as the personality of the therapist" (Schore, 2014, p. 391).

Experiential Unity model, through a right brain orientation, is a blend of talk therapy and somatic engagement of the client that is rooted in an understanding of psychobiological processes. Annette Shore, in her article "Art therapy, Attachment, and the Divided Brain," recalls attending a lecture by Allan Schore where he reiterated the challenges of using language to communicate somatic experiences (Shore, 2014, p. 91). When asked how attachment reparative work is done in therapy, Dr. Schore answered "nonverbal therapies such as art therapy are coming into the public's awareness as a possible answer because they access affective states effectively" (Shore, 2014, p. 91).

In using images and metaphors for over a decade I have noted some common themes with the consistent use of visual images/metaphors in applying Experiential Unity model. I have observed how the visual images or tools, filled in with the clients' experience, encapsulate their struggle in a new way. They also give a detached perspective when looking at their present predicament.

I have also noted the impact of the tools, or visual images, to assist in bypassing defensive responses from the clients, and potential projections onto the therapists. A case in point is a Men's anger management group. During one group a client described to the group members how he had yelled at his partner last week, but he managed not to hit her or physically react. The men in the group congratulated this individual and he received a great deal of praise for his restraint. As a facilitator of the group, and the only female in a group of 12 men, I was profoundly distressed by the conversation and was thinking on my feet what might be the most powerful way to tackle the condoning of abuse. I went to the board and drew a figure of a man and put a large bubble attached to his mouth. I then asked the client to recall all the comments he made and captured them in the bubble. We also drew a heart on the figure and captured all the feelings he was feeling in that moment. I then drew his partner and asked the group to fill in the feelings that she was likely feeling given the comments she experienced, and how the comments may shape her core beliefs about herself, and her ideas about the relationship. The men were a bit awestruck by the process, many men mentioned how eye opening the experience had been and that they had an increased awareness regarding the impact of verbal abuse. The drawing had confronted the men in the group and the lack of defensiveness was notable.

The visual images are also able to reflect "lived experience" of the client in terms of wider societal issues. This is critical information to reflect in the image; for instance, a client's history of racism, history of structural violence, a client experience of prejudice in a variety of forms. Also, important to note is how the lived experience has impacted the person on an emotional level. The visual images are also able to reflect intergenerational trauma and historical trauma, and how past experiences of a parent or grandparent have impacted the client. For instance, I have worked with several clients whose parents survived the holocaust and other First Nations clients whose parents were subjected to colonial policies of the residential school system imposed by the Canadian government. Research into racial trauma has made links to a range of physiological effects including hypervigilance to threat, flashbacks, nightmares, avoidance, suspiciousness, and somatic expressions such as headaches and heart palpitations. Building into the drawing the lived experience of parents and/or grandparents can deepen an understanding of what core beliefs, embodied emotion, and survival strategies have been passed on consciously or unconsciously. It also can bring awareness regarding the extent of trauma suffered by their family of origin members, and how it has impacted their lives.

Other aspects to build in may be dominant cultural mores which may have contributed to the client feeling alienated and an outsider from pervasive cultural norms. For instance, with one group, I constructed an image with a river depicting mainstream societal values and located their position in the river. Participants talked about being on the edge of the river, isolated, alone, and detached from the mainstream and a value system that was alienating to them. We then brainstormed the "outsider" experience, the emotional impact, what are some of the thoughts and stories that they have developed over time re their experience of being detached from mainstream society. All these experiences are built into the visual images, the goal of the visual image, metaphor or tool is to reflect at a very deep level the lived experience of the client, including all aspects of their lives.

Another key aspect of the visuals in Experiential Unity model is to assist the client in building tolerance for feelings. Many clients with a trauma history struggle to articulate their feelings, and their feeling vocabulary can be limited. With each drawing a great deal of time is taken to brainstorm the feelings that relate to the situation described. Clients often need time to locate both sensation and feelings in their body and need time to reflect on the nuances of their experience. Feelings are generally captured in the drawing by a heart on the figure with an arrow on the blank page listing as many feelings as possible. See the drawings in the text for examples of lists of feelings. This is a strong feature of the images; once feelings are ascertained clients often stare at them on the page, they appear mesmerized by the drawings. A common response is that it is very helpful to be able to see the full picture, including all their feelings related to the situation with all other aspects built in. The feelings are most often the embodied emotion that has been trapped in their body. The drawings provide an outlet to tolerate feelings that may have been suppressed historically. This is a significant strength of this model, and I believe assists in facilitating the change process. In an article, "Staying with the Metaphor," the authors Goldberg and Stephenson (2016) describe using metaphors to release and express feelings in grief work, "The power in staying with the metaphor to explore and make meaning with emotions lies not only in the abstractness or symbolic nature of the metaphor, but rather, the metaphor can be used to bring physically embodied recollections to the forefront. Furthermore, the exploration and use of metaphors is applicable to grief counseling as an intervention to promote loss adaptation and meaning making for clients grieving" (Goldberg & Stephenson, 2016, p. 105).

The other key piece I have noted in the last decade of working with images and metaphors is they assist the client stay within their window of tolerance. It is rare in my experience that the client is activated through the drawing process; I have noted this in both Experiential Unity model individual and group therapy sessions. My assumption is the detachment in the drawing process and the co-construction help provide protection from reliving the trauma and re-traumatization. In a chapter of *Metaphor as Heroic Mediator*, Wise and Nash (2013) state:

> Developing a safe environment for the essential containment of affect and memory may require approaching trauma work within a multi-dimensional framework. The metaphor provides a powerful tool to do just this . . . . Engaging metaphor as the mediator between the devastating sensorial bodily memory of trauma and the explicit narrative of *what happened* allows opportunities for bridging between fragmented parts of the self to occur. . . . Working within the metaphor can engender prospects for distancing, expansion of possibilities and explorations of meaning. Moreover, to leap directly from the sensorial to the cognitive may bypass necessary transformative work which lends substance to true healing. (Wise & Nash, 2013, pp. 99–100)

Another anecdotal aspect of the visual drawings I have noted personally is that, as a therapist, I seem to have protection from vicarious traumatization. I have observed over a 14-year period how working with drawings and visual images has shielded me from being impacted significantly or being triggered. Some of the topics I would expect to be triggering, and yet at the end of the session I have not felt drained or activated, it appears to offer a container for both client and therapist.

Another key aspect of the drawings is co-creation, collaboration, and situating the client as the expert of their experience. Each tool is most often unique for that group or individual at that time. This heightens the relevancy of the tool and the client benefits from a process that is specifically designed for them at that moment in their therapeutic process. Another aspect is the clinician attuning, supporting, and facilitating processing of traumatic material and enquiring with questions that elucidate as much of the clients experience as possible. This bottom-up processing whereby the client is teaching the clinician about their somatic experience is empowering, gives control to the client, and is congruent with a trauma-informed practice model of therapeutic engagement. This I believe also is part of the hope installation that the drawings offer, the clients are fully engaged in creating their therapy, and they leave with the therapeutic process in a concrete form, not just what they remember from the session. Clients have spoken frequently of the benefit of having the drawing with them in between sessions. One client stated that she pasted all the drawings on her ceiling and, as soon as she woke up in the morning, she felt they were there to help her get through the day and move forward. In individual sessions I make mention to the client that the drawings are like maps, and that they can keep adding to them during the week as relevant information crops up. This has inspired clients to keep their therapy active in between sessions, and again puts them in the driver seat of creating the change they are hoping to experience in their future. It also impacts how often they need to see their therapist; most clients on my caseload I see monthly. I believe this is due to the active role that the drawing creates in the interim period between sessions. Clients have also remarked how the drawings remind them of choice at times when a trauma response persuades them that there is no way out. This helps them reduce the impact of nervous system dysregulation.

In a group setting, the clients play a powerful role in creating the drawings. This facilitates an increase in group bonding, group trust, and group cohesion. The clients are actively creating and receiving the benefit of the therapeutic process they are involved in and they can see how their contribution is directly helping others in a concrete way. It also reduces dependence on the therapist, they experience the process as teamwork, and they are all making a valuable contribution.

Clients in an open crisis stabilization group in a psychiatric group therapy program were asked if they wished to give feedback anonymously regarding the tools, or visual drawings, for a potential future book. Eight clients gave feedback:

Client A: I would never have been able to learn how to survive or tolerate my depression without the tools. I refer to all of the tools because just one is not enough. I cannot stress how much better I have felt about myself since starting this particular group session. Thank you, thank you, and thank you.

Client B: Yes, I think the tools are helpful and beneficial.

1. Subject is expressed by the group during discussion, so always relevant.
2. Designed to be interactive with participants—thought provoking.
3. New—tool being copied to keep for future reference.

Client C:

1. Help me build strength when I'm feeling weak.
2. Create awareness of behavior patterns combining thoughts and tools to empower us to know we can change the way we think and see things.
3. Give us hope to know we can live a happy and peaceful life.

4. The tools are created in a sharing environment where we find we are not alone and there are others who also struggle.

Client D:

1. Collective effort.
2. Achieving positive outcome.
3. Problem solving.
4. Giving new awareness.
5. Understanding problems in objectivity.

Client E: Why the tools are helpful:

1. Provide visual metaphors/analogies for abstract concepts.
2. Accessible images are easily accessed.
3. Provide something to "grab on to." Pulling out a tool—suddenly brings me to that space of self-awareness and reminds me that I have options and choices in my reactions/responses to situations. Give me breathing space.
4. Concepts of "tools" and "tool belt" accentuate the ideas of building, rebuilding, and strengthening oneself.

Client F:

1. Great reference—I look back on them sometimes when I am journaling and they help remind me of some of the choices I can make.
2. Some of the examples really click with me and help me to make senses of my feelings—they are very visual.
3. They also remind me of where I want to go in terms of my self-growth and consequently remind me of the positive changes I've made.

Client G:

1. Tool—breathing. Why? Helps me calm myself when I feel myself becoming anxious under pressure.
2. Setting boundaries. Why? Not feeling as bad before when saying no.
3. Realizing what is important and how not to make things worse.

The visual drawings are adaptive to remote counseling or counseling on Zoom. In both situations the client can complete the drawing with guidance from the clinician or the drawing can be done together using the Zoom whiteboard. In the case of phone counseling the clinician can ask pertinent questions to draw the theme from the client and make suggestions for the drawing to fully reflect the complexity of the client's current situation.

An important component of the visual drawings is that each aspect of the drawing should be transcribed in a different color ink. This helps to distinguish the range of differing viewpoints built into the image—for instance, the impact of the situation, or next steps on dealing with the situation in different color inks. The visuals in the next section have a series of questions that can be asked, the set of answers to each question could all be recorded on the visual in a different ink color. Clients have commented over the years that the visuals help them to focus, highlight "what is" and what "isn't working," and alert them to actions they can take that will help them tackle the predicament they find themselves in.

Experiential Unity Model and Format for Individual Therapy Sessions

Steps for Therapeutic Process—Brief Version for Clients Able to Access Embodied Emotion

Step 1—Breathing/Visualization/Tapping/Body postures/Mind-Body techniques —use techniques that client feels soothes and calms his/her body.

Step 2—Breathe and feel—to identify where tension/sensation /urges are held in the body, breathe into this area, and see if a feeling can be identified. Identify as many feelings in this area as possible. Enquire regarding what the feeling may relate to if known. Clinician is attuning to information from their own body, sensing and intuiting along with the client.

Step 3—Client process regarding feelings identified and/or topic articulated regarding what experience the feelings may relate to. If the client is not wanting to address the issues that have surfaced, the client then talks about another issue of concern. Periodically check in with the body and breathe and feel, identify feelings, mutual attunement regarding need for resourcing—stopping the session and resourcing when client activation is increasing. Once a main theme has been identified client and clinician imagine a drawing that would fit the theme. For instance, feeling out of control—may be flying a flimsy aircraft with currents and intense winds creating a great deal of turbulence. Fill in drawing—capturing the present situation fully, brainstorming what else is impacting the situation, perhaps weather up ahead as an indicator of future stressors, any historical experiences that relate to this image. When one has fleshed out the image fully what will help to sturdy the plane (essentially what can one do to improve the situation)? Build in any other empowerment strategies. See drawings in text to develop ideas of how to flesh out the drawings fully, questions to ask, angles to explore, and how to build in coping strategies.

Step 4—Use clearing technique to release emotion related to past traumatic experience —tapping, breathing, visualization, movement, among others—whatever is the clients preferred clearing technique.

Step 5—Wrap up—what stood out and end with a calming technique and /or visualization for empowerment related to the drawing. Give the drawing to the client to reflect on and add to at home. Client can use it as a map to work through trauma that has surfaced or continues to surface and ease nervous system dysregulation.

Expanded Version for Each Step in Individual Counseling Which Includes Clients Too Activated to Access Embodied Emotion

Step 1—Engage in a mind/body technique that assists in calming and grounding the client. In the first session it is critical to establish a technique that assists the client in connecting with sensation/tension/urges in the body and with implicit memory. This technique is important too for calming the client when activated and outside their window of tolerance as well. For example, mindfulness, visualization, grounding, breathwork, or any other mind/body technique such as rocking back and forth, a butterfly hug by holding each opposite shoulder, squeezing stress balls, using the 5-4-3-2-1 technique naming 5 things you can see, 4 things you can feel, 3 things you can hear, 2 things you can smell, and 1 thing you can taste (balancing for dual awareness), movement, Kundalini yoga poses, hand on the heart and breathe through the hand, and using tapping in various points are some techniques that a client can explore with the clinician. Other techniques that help release oxytocin, "oxytocin is a powerful helper in the process of maintaining equanimity and can be thought of as the neurochemical foundation of resilience. Researchers have demonstrated that a single exposure to oxytocin can create a lifelong change in the brain" (Graham, 2013, p. 210). Some other ideas for an oxytocin release according to Graham are a 2-minute head rub, rubbing the back of your skull where the top of your neck meets the skull, and a 20-second body hug with someone in their life with whom they feel a sense of safety. Also recalling someone we love and have felt loved by can stimulate an oxytocin release or visualizing a spiritual figure that one has felt nurtured by. "In evoking a memory or image of feeling loved and cherished, we activate the prefrontal cortex, which triggers the hippocampus to search for explicit memories of moments when we have been held, soothed, protected, encouraged, believed in, times when we have reached out for help and received comfort and support" (Graham, 2013, p. 215).

Another key piece in the first session is to take some time to inform the client how a trauma-informed counseling session is different from other forms of individual counseling. Key pieces to discuss are:

• Time will be taken in the session to engage the body and connect with sensations as a way of knowing and embodied emotion, if the client is willing and feels comfortable to do this. Some clients may be overwhelmed because of a fear of body sensation and connecting internally. "They still don't have the experience that they're able to actually move through negative sensations into more positive sensations" (Bowen et al., 2008a, p. 6). If the client is willing to explore connection with their body this will be done by assisting the client in "noticing what they notice," and "feeling what they are feeling" including sensation and tension in the body. The client is asked if there is a particular area in their body where they feel sensation or tension, and if so to sit with the sensation and see if there is a feeling there. The client is asked if they can name a feeling, or several feelings related to the area of tension or sensation.

- A key piece to establish at the first session is finding out what helps to calm, soothe, and ground the person's body. Taking time to practice some techniques to establish what works for them is important. Also educating the client about activation and exploring the clients experience of moving outside their window of tolerance, what are some signs of activation? Alerting the client that throughout the session there will be mini breaks, if necessary, to resource their body to stay within their capacity to work with nervous system dysregulation.

- One of the biggest adjustments for clients in a trauma-informed practice session is to work at letting go of all the details of distressing situations. When a situation is overwhelming, there can be a tendency to go through all the details in a desperate attempt to release the distress or make sense of what happened. I mention to clients that I will be stopping them if they start to engage a lot of details, and we will focus on resourcing at that moment to calm their body. I point out that their body is likely reliving the event by a fully detailed account, and that there is strong likelihood they will leave the session activated, potentially feeling worse than when they came into the session. To reinforce this point I often say, "reflect on how many times you have told the 'story' and still the distress related to it hasn't changed."

- In a trauma-informed practice therapy session, it is also key to remind the client that an emphasis will be put on clearing techniques. Explaining to the client that this will assist in releasing emotion and regulating the nervous system. Many therapy sessions spend a great deal of time on problem exploration and solutions and leave out the engagement of the body in a clearing process. Given trauma has impacted the body, and its impact is held in the body, it is key to clear it from the body through a process that is beyond words. This will assist the client in experiencing shifts in the therapeutic process. Often clients report feeling lighter, clearer, and more motivated after a session where significant clearing has occurred, others experience shifts in a variety of ways, for instance, feeling more grounded or more connected with their bodies. Many clients have reported that experiencing shifts in the session is a key piece in feeling hopeful about therapy. Clearing techniques may be different for different clients, for example, for some visualizations may be powerful. A client I worked with recently had experienced a crisis of identity at a young age, a visualization included going back to that time and giving something to the young child that would help them manage the moment differently. Another visualization could be when a client connects with a family member who was abusive in their past, they could imagine themselves being protected by a white veil or contained and protected in a cylinder of safety. Visualizations can be a way of reworking the past from an empowered point of view. Other clearing techniques include tapping, movement, shaking, acupressure, or using breathwork to release the area of tension or trapped emotion. Again, it is key to find out what works and is comfortable for the client.

- A last piece to add to a trauma-informed session using Experiential Unity model is to let the client know that once we have gained an understanding of their present struggle we will capture their process in a drawing. I explain that most of the impact of trauma is held in the unconscious and that one way of accessing the unconscious and bypassing the left brain and analytical mind is to draw. This aligns with the right-to-right brain orientation mentioned in chapter 2. I also let them know that a visual offers a bridge between the prefrontal cortex and the limbic system critical for the healing process. The client can draw the drawing themselves, or if they prefer I will construct it and ask questions to help fill in the important aspects of their current situation.

Step 2—Breathe and feel—if the client can identify where tension/sensation is held in the body and breathe into this area. Sit with the sensation for a while and put your entire focus on that area of the body. Also intuit whether a feeling can be identified. Identify as many feelings in this area as possible. Answer the question: Do you have a sense of what the feeling or feelings relate to?

If the client is too activated, fearful, disassociates, or feels overwhelmed to connect with their body a step two could be grounding and calming. Then, when the client is calmer, focus on a drawing which is away from body sensation but still engages the body and captures their present moment experience. Alternatively, if the client can engage their body a little it may be helpful to practice titration as they briefly describe their present struggle. The titration process is slow and tentative, according to Levine "you just titrate the experience to the smallest amounts. And as you do this, so they have one experience here, just a tiny little experience where things were tolerable, and then a little bit later something else comes up, and you bring their attention to their bodies again. And there's another little, tiny bit of experience there. And then another one, little, tiny thing. And then pretty soon they kind of merge together, and they have some bit of a stable mass to give them refuge in the torrential sea of trauma" (Bowen et al., 2008a, p. 6).

If a client can move into step two and gain access to their body's sensations and feelings, the process can assist capturing whether any implicit memory is surfacing in their body at that moment in time. Quite often the feelings that arise initially are anxiety, anger, stress, and agitation, for example. I let the client know these feelings often sit on the surface (I call them umbrella feelings) and ask the client to imagine breathing beneath the umbrella feeling that they have stated. The individual clients I have worked with often reinforce the idea that feelings are experienced in layers. They sense that some feelings are more on the surface and that more painful feelings lie at a deeper level. Many clients have noted too that the same feeling keeps arising in their life repeatedly, but at a different level of intensity. The "entire sequence of experiences, from the embedding of traumas to the arising of implicit sensations to our deepening sensitivity to and trust of them to our openness to receiving disconfirmation, speaks again of the depth of embodied wisdom that permeates the encoding, retrieval, and healing of implicit memory. This unfolding process is also guided by the inherent wisdom of our embodied brain's innate movement toward greater integration (Siegel, 2015b), not in a reliable, predictable, left-centric way, but in the messy, tentative, unpredictable manner that is the hallmark of right-centric processes" (Badenoch, 2018, p. 174).

In Experiential Unity model, like other somatically oriented modalities, the clinician is using their own body to attune to the client's present moment experience. For example, Sensorimotor psychotherapy, Somatic experiencing, and Whole body focusing are some models that require the clinician to use their own body as a gauge of what may be happening on a somatic level with their client. Prior to a counseling session I am conscious of the need to clear any activation from my body and move into as calm and present state as possible. Developing an array of techniques that assist one's own body to ground, calm, and settle is a key habit to develop when offering trauma-informed practice counseling sessions. Personally, I find tapping very helpful to clear, but also use breathwork, movement, and few Kundalini yoga poses (those mentioned in the Kundalini yoga section) to restore my body to as full a presence as possible. Consciously or unconsciously as soon as I am in the same space as the client, I am picking up my own body sensation and attuning to the client's body, what they are saying, how they are saying it, and noting micro-movements in their body while talking. Janina Fisher, psychotherapist, consultant, and trainer in Sensorimotor psychotherapy, talks about engaging and noting her own body reactions "As I am mirroring the client's movements, or trying out what the client is trying out, I'm tracking my own body for what it feels like, knowing of course it might not be identical, but as much as possible using my own body to inform me about what's going on in the client's body. And that's one of the ways that I can maintain attunement" (Bowen et al., 2008b, p. 2). Peter Levine (founder of Somatic experiencing) supports this concept of using one's own body for information "so being able to see the body, and also being able to feel in your own body, in your own organism, the effect that this has on you, gives you a tremendous amount of information" (Bowen et al., 2008b, p. 2). Bonnie Badenoch explores the contrast in relational engagement from the left brain and right brain orientations. She states a left brain orientation involves one person needing "to do something to or for another" in contrast to a right brain orientation which "attends to our bodies, we may notice our muscles, bellies, throats and perhaps other areas respond in distinct ways when we move into this mode of relating" (Badenoch, 2018, p. 200).

It is worth noting when a client's somatic experience has been validated, fleshed out fully in a drawing and the process has also built-in choices around "what the next step may be," there is often noticeable growth by the next session in a wide range of indicators of client progress. I have noted increased motivation, increased sense of empowerment, the client is more willing to connect to feelings and identify them, clients report feeling lighter and more able to accomplish healthy risk-taking behaviours and increase their assertiveness.

Step 3—Client identifies feeling, or feelings, and topic regarding what the feelings relate to if possible. Learning to define *emotion* in a more nuanced way, being as specific as possible, a term coined by Lisa Feldman Barrett (2017) as *granularity of emotion*, is an important skill in trauma work. "Research on 'emotional granularity' or 'differentiation' supports the idea that it is a type of emotional intelligence that can improve long-term health and well-being. More fine-tuned expression of emotions is also associated with better social and emotional functioning overall" (Greenberg, 2019).

Once a specific feeling has been identified, a visual image, or metaphor, is then co-created or imagined by the clinician and discussed with the client. Essentially a question I use quite often is "When you are reflecting on the experience of feeling 'insert feeling here' does an image come to mind?" While the client is reflecting the clinician is also pondering what image may be a fit for the situation; if the client does not have an image the clinician tentatively offers an idea for the image, if neither client nor clinician has an image it is then a back-and-forth discussion around co-creating an image that fits.

For example, perhaps the client felt constriction in the throat area. He /she breathed into that area of the body and the feeling identified in the throat was "unlovable." The client may have identified that the feeling of being unlovable relates to needing to help others to be accepted. The other feelings that could emerge with unlovable are unseen, invisible, used, resentful for having to give to be accepted, that I am not lovable just for being me, regardless of whether I give or not. If the client can name a feeling but is unsure what it relates to, then an image is intuited from their experience of that feeling. This process is a right-to-right brain orientation from the clinician's and client's engagement. The process is moving into the realm of imagining, when imagination is involved, there is no "right" drawing, the process is not trying to discover what is the best metaphor or image to depict the situation, rather what image or metaphor will resonate with the client's experience. In essence it is a process of surrendering to the present moment, giving over to one's imagination, and being willing to experience some degree of vulnerability in letting go of an expert role, and rather aligning with the client in a process of co-creating. Often when I am teaching my model in workshops the barriers to learning to co-create in the moment are often impacted by a struggle to trust oneself, and a need to "get it right" and some influence of perfectionism. John Heider's quote is a good reminder of the process of a right brain orientation and the quality of surrender that is helpful. The quote is from his book Tao of Leadership titled "Knowing what is happening":

> When you cannot see what is happening do not stare harder. Relax and look gently with your inner eye. When you do not understand what a person is saying, do not grasp every word. Give up your efforts. Become silent inside and listen with your deepest self. When you are puzzled by what you see and hear, do not strive to figure things out. Stand back for a moment and become calm. When a person is calm, complex events appear simple. To know what is happening, push less, open out and be aware. See without staring. Listen quietly rather than listening hard. Use intuition and reflection rather than trying to figure things out. The more you let go of trying, and the more open and receptive you become, the more easily you will know what is happening. Also, stay in the present. (Heider, 2014, p. 27)

Once an image has been ascertained the first task with the image, or metaphor, is for it to reflect as much as possible the complexity of the client's current experience. The struggle, challenge, or problem needs to be fully fleshed out and reflect as many different angles as possible before a solution in the form of choices, or next steps, is built into the drawing. For example, with the experience of feeling "unlovable" an image that may fit could be hanging your head down and looking mainly at the ground or curled in the corner, and no one noticing that one is in the corner all hunched up. Another image that may fit could be all these outstretched hands needing something, but none of them make eye contact and the person is not seen, only as a source of giving and filling others' needs. To bring this example alive let's run with the last image of the client being surrounded by outstretched hands symbolizing need and none of the figures making eye contact. The following questions could help add information to the drawing—with each answer it is key to include the information in the drawing (See drawing 1.16 on page 100).

Some questions to ask could be:

- Who are the people with the outstretched hands lets name them, what are they wanting?
- Are some of the hands harder to set boundaries with, why is that? What is the dynamic of these relationships?
- What are some of the characteristics of these people with outstretched hands, why are they unable to see you and acknowledge your needs?
- When did you first feel this feeling of being "unlovable" and only worthy if you are giving? If it started in your family of origin, what was happening in your family at that time that this dynamic emerged and how old were you when it first came up?
- What is the impact on your heart regarding needing to give and not being seen? What are some of the feelings you are feeling now when you see the hands and they are not able to see you, or acknowledge your needs or limits? Brainstorm as many feelings as possible.
- Put an asterisk on those feelings that you felt earlier in your life; for instance, in your childhood or at an earlier time in your life. The feelings with an asterisk are often linked to implicit memory to a time of trauma.
- Let's put a bubble over your head and capture some of the thoughts you are having regarding this situation of constantly giving and not being seen.
- Now let's put a circle around your heart to reflect any core beliefs about yourself that are relevant to this situation—write in the core beliefs.
- When you look at the drawing is there anyone in your life that does not have outstretched hands and is able to see you? What is it about that relationship that helps you to be seen, what feelings are generated when you are around them?
- What do you need regarding the outstretched hands? What would you like to say to them—capture that in a cloud? Would a veil of protection be helpful? If so, let's draw it in as a big circle around you, state what will help protect you when the outstretched hands are taking too much from your perspective?

- What can you do for yourself to give yourself steadier ground to help assert and protect yourself especially when you feel you are giving too much to people who are not able to see you?
- What gifts would you like to give to yourself that will increase the feeling of lovability whether you are giving or not?

The questions are all intent on gleaning information to develop a full picture of the clients experience right now. Each answer is added into the drawing, arrows could depict influences of the past and bricks could be put under the feet to capture what is helping to get to steadier ground where one is able to set boundaries more easily. The drawings are in essence simple, but often they capture profound information which has rarely coalesced in one image that can be looked at repeatedly.

Step 4—Once the drawing has been filled in, or before, one may oscillate between filling in the drawing or clearing depending on the level of activation, keeping the clients within their window of tolerance. Please refer to the section on the incorporation of integrative techniques and Experiential Unity model for some ideas re clearing. Some other techniques suggested by Linda Graham in *Bouncing Back* may be helpful and include the following: "Rewiring old somatic memories through a body scan" (Graham, 2013, p. 219). One technique is bringing awareness to each part of the body and with each body part bring a "compassionate, caring and acceptance to any part of it that needs comfort and ease . . . the body scan is a practice to mindfully, lovingly inhabit all parts of you, to become safely aware of every experience of your body" (Graham, 2013, p. 220). A similar technique that Graham suggests for rewiring old somatic memories includes a tension/relaxation exercise whereby one tenses and relaxes different parts of the body. An alternative exercise she suggests for rewiring negative memories is "Experiment with a very simple form of reconditioning for rewiring those body-based negative memories, based on the technique of somatic experiencing developed by Dr. Peter Levine.

1. Identify a place in your body where you might be holding a somatic memory of a trauma or something that simply feels negative or unpleasant: a churning in the stomach, a tense jaw, a tightening in your back or shoulders, Notice the physical sensations.
2. Now locate a place in your body that is not feeling any distress or trauma at all—maybe your elbow or your big toe. Notice the physical sensation of being in the window of tolerance: feeling calm, relaxed, at ease. If you are currently experiencing the body-based sensations of any trauma, this window might be quite small. Focus attention on that calm, untraumatized place in the body, steadily feeling the sensations there of ease and relaxation.

3. Now switch your attention back and forth between the physical sensations of the place in your body that is not traumatized at all, and the physical sensations of the place in the body that is holding the network of the trauma memory. When you switch between awareness of the two different body parts, you are practicing a technique called pendulation (like the pendulum of a clock swinging back and forth). It's a way for you to recondition a trauma memory through body sensations alone" (Graham, 2013, pp. 225–226).

The above somatic exercises, and those mentioned in chapter 2 on integrative techniques incorporated into Experiential Unity model, assist in the release of implicit memory of trauma in the body. They also help with releasing oxytocin and assist returning the body to a calm state, and strengthening its role in regulating the nervous system and rewiring traumatic memories held in the body.

Step 5—The final step of an individual counseling session is to do a final calming strategy that relaxes and soothes the body to reduce any activation from the session. The calming technique again could be a preferred strategy for the client or something like the bumble bee breath, if they find it helpful, which can be both grounding and calming. Also co-creating a visualization and summarize what stood out in the session. Visualizations can be a powerful way to end the session as it can be helpful in integrating the work that has been addressed in the session. According to Dr. Tara Swart, a neuroscientist, leadership coach, author, and medical doctor, "to inform your visualization, you can imagine your successes as if they already happened. Doing this allows you to tap into another powerful brain training mechanism. Simply imagining something can deliver the physical and mental benefits of the action that you desire. Studies show that people who imagine themselves flexing a muscle achieve actual physical strength gains. Why? Because they activate the same pathways in the brain that relate to the actual, real-life movement of the muscle. Sports psychologists have long since understood the value of this kind of imaginative exercise" (Swart, 2019).

Graham in *Bouncing Back* reinforces the power of the brain to support the therapeutic process. She states "evoking refuges and resources in the imagination can feel as real to the brain as having them physically present. The possibilities of using imagination to rewire our brains can stretch towards the infinite" (Graham, 2013, p. 100).

Experiential Unity model uses visualization as a way of integrating the various processes in the drawing, and to consolidate the learning and healing aspect of the drawing, as mentioned in an earlier section. The question for the clinician and client is, "What would be healing and empowering to visualize and help in the integration of the work we have just done?" For instance, going back to the example of "feeling unlovable" and only feeling worthy if one is giving excessively to others, a visualization could be remembering moments with others, or oneself, when one was able to feel lovable and accepted for who one is and not for tasks done for others. Another healing visualization could be visualizing protection against those who regularly have outstretched hands, having a shield of protection in place, may assist in asserting oneself when needed. It could be an invisible cloak or an opaque cylinder that offers protection, it could be hands or wings over the heart, or a safe place one automatically goes to where it is easier to make decisions from a clear and grounded place. Clients have often remarked how powerful the visualizations are and that they have assisted them markedly in their healing.

Examples of Visuals/Metaphors/Images/Drawings for Experiential Unity Model and Individual Counseling

An important piece to note is there is often overlap in the drawings, sometimes they are dealing with similar themes and often it is the same feelings coming up repeatedly. When I first started to do the drawings, I thought initially that a similar theme wouldn't be helpful to unpack, particularly if it dealt with the same constellation of feelings again. However, I have changed my mind wholeheartedly re this aspect, what I have come to learn is that each drawing provides an opportunity to peel back another layer of trauma. Clients have taught me over time that although the drawing is a similar theme, they are experiencing it as "healing for this moment in time" and again it helps them to experience "being seen and understood" at a deep level. They also find it helpful for internal barriers to be acknowledged and considered part of the complexity of shifting, changing, and working through past pain and trauma.

A key piece of the drawings is that it is critical to flesh out all the concerns fully, especially the impact on feelings, so they are understood at a deep level before a solution in any way is introduced into the drawing. My belief around this is that a critical piece in the change process is "to be seen and heard and understood at a deep level." When painstaking time is taken to get as full an understanding of the problem as possible, and the emotional impact, this process assists the client in their willingness to surrender to change if they are ready.

Stress/Pain Container—Connection/Disconnection

I have used this drawing in the first session of a Deepening self-connection and Healing group, a Coping with Depression Group, a Coping with Anxiety group, Mindfulness and Relaxation group, and a Self-compassion group. I

Visual 1.1 Stress/Pain Container - Connection/Disconnection

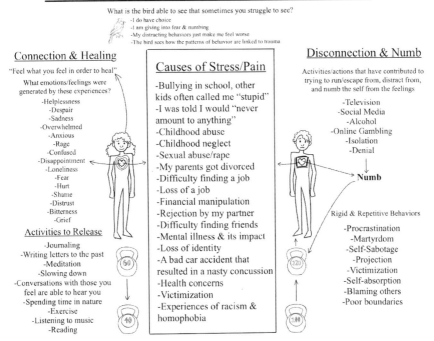

What is the bird able to see that sometimes you struggle to see?
- I do have choice
- I am giving into fear & numbing
- My distracting behaviors just make me feel worse
- The bird sees how the patterns of behavior are linked to trauma

Connection & Healing

"Feel what you feel in order to heal"

What emotions/feelings were
generated by these experiences?
- Helplessness
- Despair
- Sadness
- Overwhelmed
- Anxious
- Rage
- Confused
- Disappointment
- Loneliness
- Fear
- Hurt
- Shame
- Distrust
- Bitterness
- Grief

Activities to Release

- Journaling
- Writing letters to the past
- Meditation
- Slowing down
- Conversations with those you
feel are able to hear you
- Spending time in nature
- Exercise
- Listening to music
- Reading

Causes of Stress/Pain

- Bullying in school, other kids often called me "stupid"
- I was told I would "never amount to anything"
- Childhood abuse
- Childhood neglect
- Sexual abuse/rape
- My parents got divorced
- Difficulty finding a job
- Loss of a job
- Financial manipulation
- Rejection by my partner
- Difficulty finding friends
- Mental illness & its impact
- Loss of identity
- A bad car accident that resulted in a nasty concussion
- Health concerns
- Victimization
- Experiences of racism & homophobia

Disconnection & Numb

Activities/actions that have contributed to
trying to run/escape from, distract from,
and numb the self from the feelings
- Television
- Social Media
- Alcohol
- Online Gambling
- Isolation
- Denial

Numb

Rigid & Repetitive Behaviors
- Procrastination
- Martyrdom
- Self-Sabotage
- Projection
- Victimization
- Self-absorption
- Blaming others
- Poor boundaries

Figure 1.1   Stress Pain Container. Illustration by Brooke Kelly.

have also used it for a first session in an individual therapy session. This visual is powerful in building awareness about events that have occurred over a lifetime and contributed to traumatic memories and nervous system dysregulation. It also assists clients in becoming aware of the legacy of embodied emotion. The list of embodied emotion added to the drawing can be relevant for future sessions given some emotions reoccur regardless of the situation. The drawing can also provide insight into the impact of the client's lifestyle and how it contributes to connection or disconnection from self. It is also helpful for the client and clinician to assess the client's capacity to self-soothe and self-care, and be more aware regarding fears of feeling feelings, and also gain insight into deep-seated patterns that can be very challenging to tackle. Clients have mentioned that the drawing gives them a bird's-eye view to their situation, and that they also become more aware of how they are using numbing or distracting techniques to distance from feelings. They also have noted the long list of numbing techniques versus the often-short list of self-care and self-soothing strategies. It has also assisted them in building awareness around patterns of behavior that are a direct result of the embodied emotion, and the concept of maintaining walls around their heart that keeps them stuck. Clients also find the terms connection and release embodied emotion and disconnection and numb helpful for understanding the healing process. Other clients have mentioned that the drawing highlights choice, a way out of their present predicament, and educates them about the long-term impact of traumatic experiences and how it has been held in their body. These are just some of the insights clients have shared over the years of using this visual.

Questions to Ask to Fill in the Visual and Instructions

1. List answers to these questions in the container:
   What events have occurred in your life that have caused significant stress or pain? Reflect all the way back to childhood. Events can also include experiences such as bullying, name calling, and being told something very hurtful by someone that has stuck with you over the years and you keep reliving it at tough moments?

   In prior sessions clients talk about divorce of parents, betrayal by a partner, being called "stupid" or "they will never amount to anything" as some examples. Other events listed are childhood abuse, childhood neglect, rape, sexual abuse, financial manipulation, racism, bullying at school, rejection by partner, difficulty finding friends, homophobia, loss of a job, mental illness and its impact, loss of identity, car accident, victimization, and health concerns to name a few areas. All these events or situations are listed in the container in the client's words as much as possible. It is important to go with their phrasing as it is their way of interpreting the event or situation.

2. Draw a figure on either side of the top part of the container. Draw a heart on each figure. Put connection and healing on the left-hand side in red ink and disconnection and numb on the right-hand side in blue ink. Draw an arrow from the heart of the left figure onto the open page and fill in responses to the following question.

   What emotions/feelings were generated by these experiences? Brainstorm as many as possible putting them at the end of the arrow on the open page. Take time to reflect on the full range of feelings that would have been felt regarding the event. This list is critical as it is most often reflective of emotion that has been trapped in the body and is adding to nervous system dysregulation. Some of the feelings clients have shared include helplessness, hopelessness, despair, sadness, lost, overwhelmed, anxious, angry, rage, confused, disappointed, loneliness, uncertainty, alone, fear, hurt, shame, guilt, distrust, bitterness, and grief to name a few. I spend a long time with clients in a group setting or in an individual session looking at the events and imagining what feelings may come up. When these feelings are unacknowledged, they can create barriers to change or keep clients stuck in patterns of behavior which are hard to break. This also pays attention to the skill mentioned earlier of "granularity of emotion," whereby the client learns the skill of naming feelings with a high degree of specificity and precision. Many clients I have worked with have a limited range of words to describe their feelings, they commonly use the word stress, anxious, or overwhelmed which are generalized feelings. I ask clients to breathe beneath this umbrella or overarching feeling to see if another deeper feeling is evident.

3. On the right-hand side draw some walls around the heart of the figure on the right. Put the term Disconnection and numb over the top of the figure. Now write a list of activities or actions on the one list and patterns of behavior on a second list. Indicate each list with an arrow dropping down to the list. This list is reflective of actions and activities that have contributed to trying to run, escape, distract, and numb from the feelings. This list has often included too much television or social media scrolling, using drugs and alcohol, excess activities such as work addiction, exercise addiction, shopping or gambling addiction, constant noise, over-involvement in others' lives to distract, staying isolated, wearing a mask, denial, busyness, constantly moving, giving over to distraction regularly, and excessive coffee or sugar. The second list are patterns of behavior for example that have become rigid and repetitive in the clients life. They can include perfectionism, procrastination, martyrdom, self-sabotage, projection, victimization, blaming others, self-absorption, caretaking others, and poor boundary setting. I then ask clients "How heavy is the load in the container?" They may mention 100 pounds; I also link the heaviness to difficulties in motivation. I ask them "What is happening regarding the weight if you continue with the disconnecting activities?" Most clients realize it is getting heavier and have found the link between disconnecting behaviors and feeling weighed down and unmotivated helpful, and also encouraging for increasing connecting and healing activities.

4. On the left-hand side the figure has an open heart and the term Connection and heal is above it—I generally put an arrow from the heart with the phrase "feel what you feel in order to heal." I then ask the group "What activities do you do that assist you in releasing feelings, soothing, calming and relaxing your body?" Generally, clients I have worked with have a list of activities that calm and soothe their bodies, but most often the piece that is neglected is ways to release feelings. Some methods that are mentioned are journal writing and tapping. Writing letters can be an important strategy too (for the most part you don't send) for clients wanting to work through unresolved past relationship issues or traumatic

experiences. The letters are intended to be a release and an opportunity to state what may have not been acknowledged to date. I mention to clients this is a process and may involve writing 10 or more letters to the same person to release most of the pain. Again, I reinforce the idea with clients that releasing pain can be like peeling back an onion, once one layer is released another layer rises to the surface. Other ways of releasing feelings may include having important conversations that have felt off limits with those you feel are able to hear you. Also asking clients "What boundaries do you need to put in place to protect yourself more?"

Activities clients mention to soothe and calm their body include slowing down, meditation, spending time in nature, yoga, sharing time with friends, movement, dancing, reading a book, listening to music, and taking more time to relax.

An additional item to add to the drawing could be drawing a bird at the top of the page and asking clients "What is the bird able to see that sometimes you struggle to see?" Clients have typically mentioned that I do have choice, that I am giving into fear and numbing, that they weren't aware that the distracting behaviors were making them feel worse and blocked their healing process. They also mention the bird can see patterns of behavior linked to past trauma and challenging feelings, and that their distracting and numbing list is generally a lot longer than their connecting and healing list. Clients also mention how helpful the concept of developing a "bird's-eye view" is and how they can use that in other situations, helping them detach a bit from getting sucked into the intensity of their situation. This tool can be used periodically for clients to check in regarding their progress, and to assess the implementation of more healing strategies and a reduction in disconnection overall.

Tracking the History of Emotion Drawing

A drawing I have found particularly powerful for clients to teach them about the impact of implicit memory, and that the memory is often held in the body for decades is called "Tracking the history of emotion." It is also highly instructive in educating the client about the power of conscious, or unconscious implicit memory, to attract experiences that will trigger memories held in the body. "Neuroscientists have discovered that about 80 percent of the neural instructions for behavior are recorded in implicit memory, outside our conscious awareness" and Graham reinforces this point with "Even when we are old enough to process experiences explicitly, many are forgotten; but they remain stored in our implicit memory and affect our choices and behaviors in ways we are not aware of" (Graham, 2013, pp. 36–37).

Visual 1.2 Tracking the History of Emotion

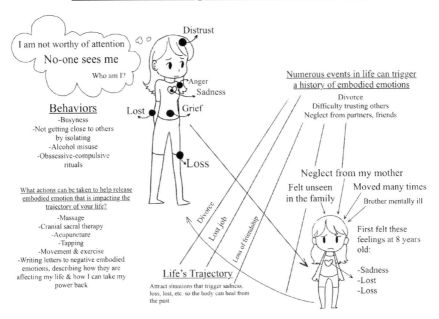

Figure 1.2 Tracking the History of Emotion. Illustration by Brooke Kelly.

"The tracking the history of emotion" drawing is helpful for clients who can connect with their bodies sensation/tension/urges and are able to work at centering and clearing to maintain their window of tolerance. Additionally, clients who have a high degree of awareness of feelings realize they are easily triggered. The exercise starts with step one and step two outlined previously. In the breathing and feeling process the client attunes to sensation/tension/urges as a way of knowing, and if possible, names a feeling they are feeling in the moment. To illuminate the process distrust as the first feeling felt will be used. Draw a body and ask the client the following questions

Some questions to use to fill in the image are;

1. Ask the client: What other feelings are present with distrust—they too are named, the feelings are represented as dots on the area of the body the client is feeling the sensation and feeling. The feelings may be distrust, sadness, lost, anger, and loss.
2. I then ask the client "When did you first feel these feelings, what age were you when you first felt some or all of these feelings?" The client most often instinctively names the age that is relevant. I have done this drawing in demonstrations of Experiential Unity model in monthly

workshops for years. To date the clients are able to name the age in seconds;, however, if not they can guess at the age.

3. Draw a stick figure representing the age they first felt the feelings. Then add the feelings felt at a younger age, it may not be all of the feelings felt in the moment. Add them to a symbolic younger body and put the age above the drawing.

4. Ask the client what situations or events were occurring in your life that contributed to these feelings. Use arrows in the direction of the head to describe what was happening at the time for this younger version of self that helps explain the feelings they were feeling. Clients often mention events like neglect from mother, mentally ill brother, felt unseen in the family, and moved many times. Other situations could include parents divorce, dealing with an alcoholic father, parents abandoned me and left me with my grandparents, my mother had a nervous breakdown, the family was in a car accident, I became ill and was bed ridden for months, I got bullied at school, I experienced racism by my teacher, my father lost his job, we had to move to another country as some examples. As many experiences are captured as possible. Once the events are fully described, the client is then asked to reflect on the feelings placed on the child-like figure and develop a timeline of when the feelings may have resurfaced at other times in life. For instance, if the child felt sadness, lost, and loss at around 8 years old due to maternal neglect, a timeline of when sadness, lost, and loss reoccurred could be at 9 years old when I was expelled from school, at 13 I left home for a while to live with a friend, at 15 I was caught shoplifting, at 21 I got pregnant and had an abortion, all these events potentially loop back to the three dominant embodied feelings related to the trauma of neglect of mother.

Developing a timeline based on the initial feelings felt in the body is powerful for a variety of reasons. Clients have remarked that it helps to see how much-embodied emotions are unconsciously impacting events in their present life. The drawing also gives a birds-eye view to their situation and explains the persistence of self-destructive patterns in their life. It has also assisted clients in paying more attention to their feelings, increasing their self-awareness of choices, and helping them link their present behavior and choices to implicit memory held in their body.

5. The drawing can also be expanded to include thoughts and core beliefs. A question to ask a client could be: When you feel these feelings what thoughts come to mind? With the feelings of sadness, lost, and loss some thoughts could be I can't trust anyone, I am confused, and if people knew me they would reject me. A bubble can be drawn over the head to write in the thoughts the client mentions. Behaviors that relate to the thoughts and feelings can be put under the feet; this reflects a foundation of a particular

lifestyle that mirrors the impact of the thoughts and feelings. Behaviors might be obsessive-compulsive rituals, drug and alcohol misuse, busyness, not getting close to others by isolating. Core beliefs can also be ascertained by reflecting on the thoughts and feelings and intuiting what core beliefs fit. With this grouping of thoughts and feelings what might be an example of a core belief? This core belief may have developed in times of trauma and then be reinforced by unhelpful patterns that consolidate the core belief. A core belief might include I am a failure, I am not enough, I'm don't know who I am, or I'm unlovable. Toward the conclusion of every drawing, it is critical to build in a remedy to the situation, or a solution of some sort, that will help reduce the entrenchment of the patterns and an overall stuck feeling.

6. Ask the client what actions they could take that would help release the embodied emotion and its impact. They could also explore some integrative modalities that appeal to them if they are open. Some ideas for releasing emotion stuck in the body could be a deep tissue massage, cranial sacral therapy, acupuncture, tapping, movement, and shaking. The client could also explore taking action that undermines some of the stuck patterns of behavior that reinforce their core beliefs and thinking.

7. Writing numerous letters to sadness, lost, and loss describing how it is affecting one's life and how one can take one's power back—a portion of these letters are often helpful to read in the next session.

Internal Conflict Drawing

Each client situation is unique and so generally I am using a new drawing each time. The drawing reflects in a specific way what the client is experiencing, with as much complexity as possible. However, themes do emerge in some clients' situations and so a drawing that maps out ambivalence, or internal conflict, may be relevant to many clients you are working with therapeutically. The feeling in the body could include conflicted, helpless, confused, or angry as some examples. I have used the internal conflict drawing for a range of areas, for instance, ambivalence about reducing drug or alcohol intake as a numbing strategy, remaining in a relationship with a partner or continuing to have contact with parents who have been abusive or unsupportive in the past. The visual has also been helpful in situations, for instance, whether to continue therapy or not, willingness to be more assertive, and mapping out ambivalence re a job. Again, with any drawing it is critical to capture as much of the complexity of the situation as possible.

Start by drawing a body with a heart on it using the example of whether to have contact with unsupportive parents.

Some questions to use to fill in the image are:

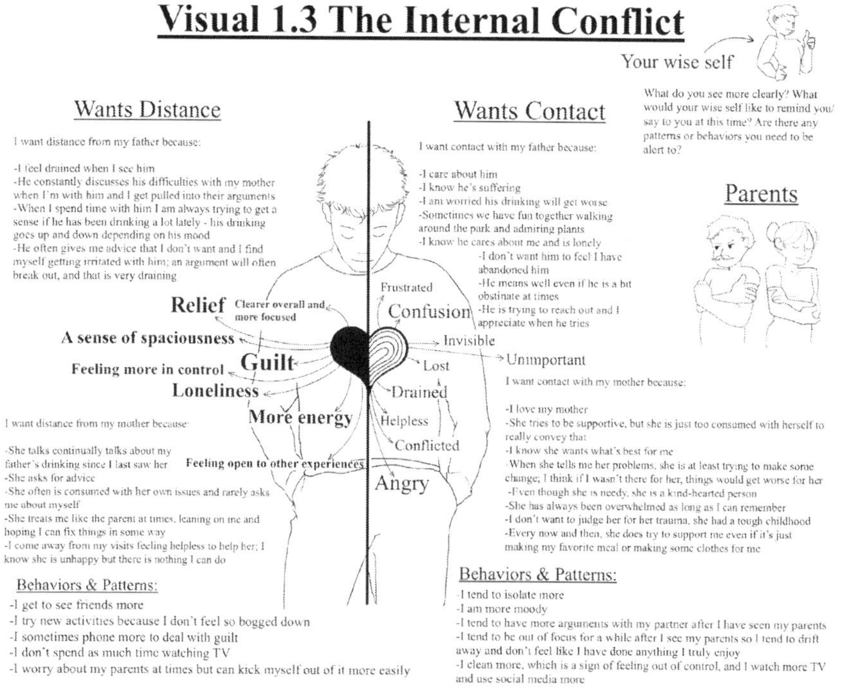

Visual 1.3 The Internal Conflict

Your wise self

What do you see more clearly? What would your wise self like to remind you/ say to you at this time? Are there any patterns or behaviors you need to be alert to?

Wants Distance

I want distance from my father because:

-I feel drained when I see him
-He constantly discusses his difficulties with my mother when I'm with him and I get pulled into their arguments
-When I spend time with him I am always trying to get a sense if he has been drinking a lot lately - his drinking goes up and down depending on his mood
-He often gives me advice that I don't want and I find myself getting irritated with him; an argument will often break out, and that is very draining

Relief Clearer overall and more focused

A sense of spaciousness

Feeling more in control **Guilt**

Loneliness

More energy

Feeling open to other experiences

I want distance from my mother because:

-She talks continually talks about my father's drinking since I last saw her
-She asks for advice
-She often is consumed with her own issues and rarely asks me about myself
-She treats me like the parent at times, leaning on me and hoping I can fix things in some way
-I come away from my visits feeling helpless to help her; I know she is unhappy but there is nothing I can do

Behaviors & Patterns:

-I get to see friends more
-I try new activities because I don't feel so bogged down
-I sometimes phone more to deal with guilt
-I don't spend as much time watching TV
-I worry about my parents at times but can kick myself out of it more easily

Wants Contact

I want contact with my father because:

-I care about him
-I know he's suffering
-I am worried his drinking will get worse
-Sometimes we have fun together walking around the park and admiring plants
-I know he cares about me and is lonely
-I don't want him to feel I have abandoned him
-He means well even if he is a bit obstinate at times
-He is trying to reach out and I appreciate when he tries

Frustrated

Confusion

Invisible

Lost → Unimportant

Drained

Helpless

Conflicted

Angry

I want contact with my mother because:

-I love my mother
-She tries to be supportive, but she is just too consumed with herself to really convey that
-I know she wants what's best for me
-When she tells me her problems, she is at least trying to make some change; I think if I wasn't there for her, things would get worse for her
-Even though she is needy, she is a kind-hearted person
-She has always been overwhelmed as long as I can remember
-I don't want to judge her for her trauma, she had a tough childhood
-Every now and then, she does try to support me even if it's just making my favorite meal or making some clothes for me

Parents

Behaviors & Patterns:

-I tend to isolate more
-I am more moody
-I tend to have more arguments with my partner after I have seen my parents
-I tend to be out of focus for a while after I see my parents so I tend to drift away and don't feel like I have done anything I truly enjoy
-I clean more, which is a sign of feeling out of control, and I watch more TV and use social media more

Figure 1.3   Internal Conflict. Illustration by Brooke Kelly.

1. When you think about the conflicting feelings re contact with parents what do you feel is the ratio of wanting contact and wanting distance? Does the drawing include both of your parents or just one of them? For the sake of the exercise let's say the client mentioned it is both my father and my mother for different reasons.

2. Let's draw a line down the body and through the heart reflecting the ratio, for instance 60/40 ratio or 70/30—then what should we call the two sides? For example, wants contact or wants distance?

3. Choose one of the sections to work on first—for example, wants distance. List all the reasons why you want distance—let's start with your father. This could include feel drained when I see him, he constantly discusses his difficulties with my mother, and I get pulled into their arguments. Also, when I spend time with him, I am trying to assess his drinking even if I don't want to—his drinking goes up and down depending on his mood. He is often giving me advice that I don't want so I get irritated with him and then an argument might start that I find draining.

4. Why do you want distance from your mother? Fill in all the details and link it to the distance side. For instance, she talks continually about my

father's drinking since I last saw her, she asks for advice, she often is consumed with her own issues and rarely asks me about myself, she treats me like the parent at times leaning on me and hoping I can fix things in some way. I come away from my visits feeling helpless to help her, I know she is unhappy but there is nothing I can do.

5. Now let's list all the reasons you do want contact starting again with your father. The example may include I care about him, I know he's suffering, I am worried his drinking will get worse, sometimes we have fun together walking around the park and admiring plants, I know he cares about me and is lonely, I don't want him to feel I have abandoned him, he means well even if he is a bit obstinate at times, he is trying to reach out and I appreciate it when he tries.

6. Now list all the reasons why you want contact with your mother. I love my mother, she tries to be supportive to me she is just too consumed with herself to really convey that, I know she wants what's best for me, when she tells me her problems she is at least trying to make some change. I think if I wasn't there for her things might get worse for her. Even though she is needy she is a kind-hearted person, she has always been overwhelmed as long as I can remember, I don't want to judge her for her trauma, she had a tough childhood. Every now and then she does try and support me even if it just making my favorite meal or making some clothes for me.

7. Now move onto the heart and put on one side of the heart the feelings that are generated by distance, they may be relief, a sense of spaciousness, guilt, loneliness, feeling more in control, clearer overall and more focused, more energy and feeling more open to other experiences. The feelings generated by contact with both parents are confusion, lost, invisible, drained, helpless, conflicted, frustrated, and angry.

8. When you reflect on feelings related to "being distant" from your parents what are some of the behaviors or patterns that are linked to those feelings? Some examples are I get to see my friends more, I try new activities because I don't feel so bogged down, I sometimes phone my parents because I feel guilty, I don't spend as much time watching TV, I do ruminate and worry about them at times but am able to kick myself out of that feeling more easily.

9. When you focus on behaviors that are often generated when you have quite a bit of contact with your parents what are they? Some ideas might include I tend to isolate more, I am more moody, I tend to have more arguments with my partner after I have seen them, I tend to be out of focus for a while after I see them, tend to drift away and I don't feel I have done anything I truly enjoy. I tend to do a lot more cleaning which

is a sign of feeling out of control, and I tend to watch a lot more TV and spend more time on social media.

To add to the drawing and get a detached perspective you could add a symbol of "your wise self." From the figure at the top representing "a wise self" the following questions may be pertinent:

a) When you look over the drawing what are your observations—what do you see more clearly? What would your wise self like to remind you of and say to you at this time?

b) Are there any patterns of behavior you need to be alert to?

c) What are your choices with regard to connecting or distancing from your parents?

d) When you make a more unhelpful choice, what are your thoughts and feelings that encourage you to acquiesce your boundaries even if you don't want to?

e) Given life is constantly in flux, which choice would you prefer to make most of the time and why, and under what circumstances?

f) Is there any strategy or clearing technique you would like to practice more to help you clear intense feelings?

g) Is there a letter you could write to your father or mother or both to explore more fully the impact on you when you have contact? In the letter you could also write out some boundaries you may need in the future to protect yourself. Most often it is helpful not to send it unless one has trust in their capacity to hear one's pain fully.

Victimization and Giving Up versus Choice

This visual is very powerful for a client feeling stuck and mired in behaviors and patterns that are contributing to them feeling overwhelmed, immobilized, and victimized by life. The feeling in the body may be stuck, helpless, hopeless, despair to name a few. The stuck feeling is represented by a swamp, client or clinician draws a swamp-like image and draws a body in the swamp, now an arrow with "giving up" at the end of it goes from the swamp to the open page.

Some questions to use to fill in the image are:

1. What feelings are generated by this experience of living life as if you are in a swamp right now? The list of feelings a client may state could be anger, self-loathing, confusion, lost, victimized, self-pity, hurt, misunderstood, disorientation, bewilderment, overwhelmed, depressed, anxious, shame, guilt, and self-rejection.

Visual 1.4 Victimization and Giving up Versus Choice

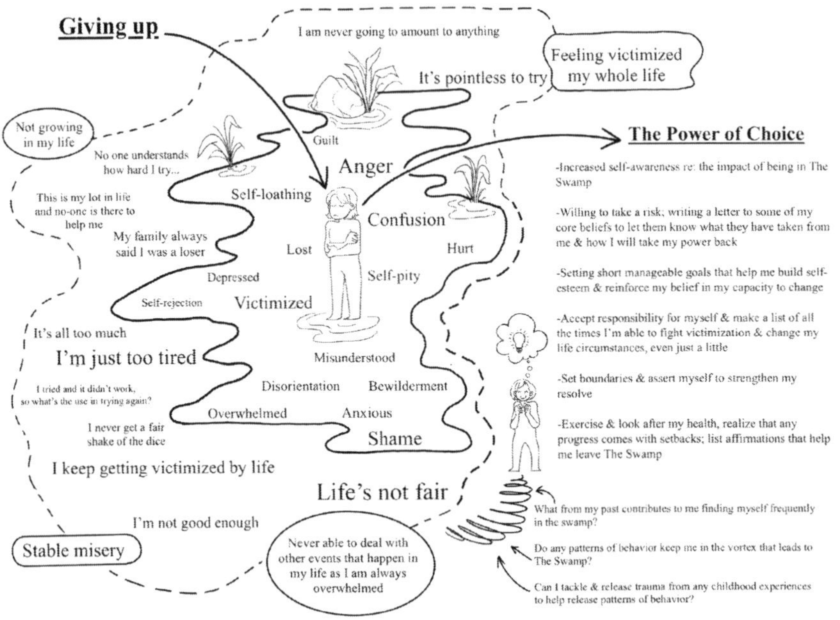

Figure 1.4 **Victimization and Giving Up versus Choice.** Illustration by Brooke Kelly.

2. The next step is to brainstorm with the client what thoughts and core beliefs contribute to you remaining in the swamp and struggling to get out. Use arrows pointing to the swamp and name each arrow with a thought or core belief or capture them in an external layer of swamp. The thoughts and core beliefs mentioned could include it's pointless to try, I am never going to amount to anything, my family always said I was a loser, I tried and it didn't work so what's the use in trying again, I'm just too tired, I keep getting victimized by life, no one understands how hard I try, it's all too much, life's not fair, I never get a fair shake of the dice, I'm not good enough, this is my lot in life, and no one is there to help me as some examples.

3. The next question to ask could be: What is the consequence on your life of remaining in the swamp long term? This could be indicated by outer circles near the swamp indicating the future. The consequence could be not growing in my life, feeling victimized my whole life, never being able to deal with other events that happen in my life as am always overwhelmed, stable misery, and an ongoing feeling of victimization.

4. Now the impact has been fleshed out fully, the next piece is to ask the client if they are willing to explore a process that might help in eventually

leaving the swamp. If the client is in agreement, then an arrow named the "power of choice" is drawn from the swamp to an open page. All the steps in the process are transcribed, they could include the following: increased self-awareness re the impact of being in the swamp, willing to take a risk, writing a letter to some of my core beliefs and letting them know what they have taken from me, and also how I will take my power back. Setting short manageable goals that help to build self-esteem and that reinforce my belief in my capacity to change. Accept responsibility for myself, make a list of all the times I am able to fight victimization and change my life circumstance, even if it's a little bit. Set boundaries and assert myself to strengthen my resolve. Exercise, look after my health and realize that any progress comes with setbacks, list some affirmations that will help with my efforts out of the swamp.

5. The last question may be: Is there any issue I need to work through from my past which contributes to finding myself frequently in the swamp? This could be reflected by a vortex that spirals from the feet of the body down in a spiral. What feelings and behaviors are reflective of being in the vortex? Are there any childhood issues that are triggered in the vortex? Do any patterns of behavior keep me in the vortex? What helps to slowly rise from the vortex step by step? Can I process unintegrated emotions from any traumatic childhood experiences that keep me stuck?

Dealing with Turbulence in Life

This is another common theme for clients. The feeling in the body that may represent this visual may be out of control, fear, confused, uncertainty, and helpless as some examples. The turbulence could be represented by a river with eddies, whirlpools, and large boulders in the river. The client could be placed in a small raft on the river heading in one direction facing boulders and turbulence represented by the whirlpools and eddies in the river.

Some questions to use to fill in the image are:

1. What are the whirlpools, eddies, and boulders in your life? The whirlpools and eddies may be not being able to manage my work demands, not keeping up with commitments, having to deal with conflict situations at work or home, lack of time, and others incessant demands, for example. Sometimes eddies and whirlpools can take us into a spiraling vortex. This often is symbolic of situations that trigger unresolved family of origin issues. It may be a conflict with a work colleague triggering unresolved parental issues so the intensity of the situation is felt deeply. It could be helpful to indicate whether any of the eddies or whirlpools link to family of origin issues. The boulders in the river could be situations

Visual 1.5 Dealing with Turbulence in Life

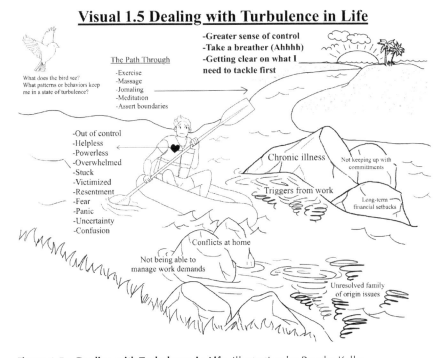

The Path Through
-Exercise
-Massage
-Jornaling
-Meditation
-Assert boundaries

-Greater sense of control
-Take a breather (Ahhhh)
-Getting clear on what I need to tackle first

What does the bird see?
What patterns or behaviors keep me in a state of turbulence?

-Out of control
-Helpless
-Powerless
-Overwhelmed
-Stuck
-Victimized
-Resentment
-Fear
-Panic
-Uncertainty
-Confusion

Chronic illness

Not keeping up with commitments

Triggers from work

Long-term financial setbacks

Conflicts at home

Not being able to manage work demands

Unresolved family of origin issues

Figure 1.5   Dealing with Turbulence in Life. Illustration by Brooke Kelly.

that are immovable in life, and where one has to work at acceptance of "what is." It could be an illness or financial circumstances that are not going to change in the near future, for example. Anything the client is experiencing that feels outside their capacity to change it.

2. Once the whirlpools, eddies, and boulders are named a next step could be to draw a heart on the figure in the boat. Then list all the feelings the person is feeling by facing these current circumstances. A list of feelings may include out of control, stuck, helpless, powerless, overwhelmed, victimized, resentment, self-doubt, frustration, uncertainty, fear, panic, and confusion as some examples. Again, from a trauma-informed perspective it is key to spend as much time on listing feelings as possible as this is reflective of embodied emotion related to trauma, which is likely contributing to the client feeling triggered in their present circumstance.

3. The next step in filling out the image could be imagining a beach up ahead. Drawing in a beach up ahead, no matter how small it appears to the client in the boat, and asking:

If you were able to get to a beach even for a short while what would you experience on the beach? How would you know you have arrived there? The client might state I will feel a greater sense of control, I could take a breather, getting clearer on what I need to tackle first as some examples.

4. Draw a path from the boat to the beach and name it "the path through." Brainstorm with the client: What are all the actions you can take that will help you get to the path through so you can access the beach? The client may start listing a range of healthcare strategies like exercise, go for a massage, spend some time journal writing and release feelings, meditation, assert self, and set boundaries for instance.

5. Add a bird at the top of the picture and ask the client: What does the bird see? Is there anything you can do on a regular basis to lessen the turbulence? Is there a pattern of behavior that increases turbulence in your life? Can you take any action that will undermine the pattern? What embodied emotion keeps surfacing with this pattern—What helps you to release embodied emotion? Can you write a letter to these emotions so you can drain their impact?

How to Reclaim Your Brain and Create New Patterns

This visual is very helpful in educating clients about past trauma, its impact, the importance of building awareness regarding unhelpful thoughts, core beliefs, and embodied emotion that undermine progress. It also increases awareness of the importance of developing new neural pathways and what helps to do that, and the visual can help clients adjust their expectations of timely progress given the complex factors that influence the process of change. Start the process by drawing a body on the center page. On the top of the head of the figure draw dizzying circles around the head depicting the impact of unhelpful messages.

Some questions to use to fill in the image are:

1. What are some unhelpful thoughts and beliefs about yourself that keep coming up? Put a line from the head to the open page to capture each thought and core belief. Some examples could be I'm a victim, I will never amount to anything, I'm not good enough, I don't have the strength to deal with my problems, I'm a loser, nothing I do will make a difference, what's the point in trying, no one gets me, I'm unlovable, nobody seems to care about how I feel. Now draw a house on the left-hand side of the drawing and call it childhood home.

2. Ask the client to put an asterisk next to the thoughts and core beliefs that link back to childhood, also put a line linking them to the childhood home. Under the childhood home put behaviors that were adaptive then but are likely unhelpful now. If applicable help the client make the link between these behaviors and unhelpful neural pathways. Some of

Visual 1.6 How to Reclaim the Brain and Create new Patterns

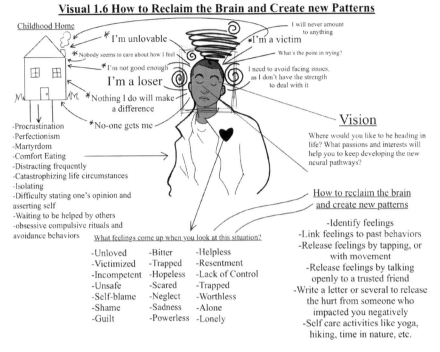

Childhood Home

I'm unlovable
Nobody seems to care about how I feel
I'm not good enough
I'm a loser
Nothing I do will make a difference
No-one gets me

I will never amount to anything
I'm a victim
What's the point in trying?
I need to avoid facing issues, as I don't have the strength to deal with it

-Procrastination
-Perfectionism
-Martyrdom
-Comfort Eating
-Distracting frequently
-Catastrophizing life circumstances
-Isolating
-Difficulty stating one's opinion and asserting self
-Waiting to be helped by others
-obsessive compulsive rituals and avoidance behaviors

Vision

Where would you like to be heading in life? What passions and interests will help you to keep developing the new neural pathways?

How to reclaim the brain and create new patterns

-Identify feelings
-Link feelings to past behaviors
-Release feelings by tapping, or with movement
-Release feelings by talking openly to a trusted friend
-Write a letter or several to release the hurt from someone who impacted you negatively
-Self care activities like yoga, hiking, time in nature, etc.

What feelings come up when you look at this situation?

-Unloved	-Bitter	-Helpless
-Victimized	-Trapped	-Resentment
-Incompetent	-Hopeless	-Lack of Control
-Unsafe	-Scared	-Trapped
-Self-blame	-Neglect	-Worthless
-Shame	-Sadness	-Alone
-Guilt	-Powerless	-Lonely

Figure 1.6   How to Reclaim the Brain and Create New Patterns. Illustration by Brooke Kelly.

these behaviors could be procrastination, perfectionism, martyrdom, comfort eating, distracting frequently, catastrophizing life circumstances, isolating, difficulty stating one's opinion and asserting self, waiting to be helped by others, obsessive-compulsive rituals, and avoidance behaviors.

3. Ask the client: When they look at this situation what feelings come up? Write the list of feelings and link them to the heart. The feelings could include unloved, victimized, incompetent, unsafe, self-blame, shame, guilt, bitter, trapped, hopeless, scared, neglect, sadness, powerless, helpless, resentment, lack of control, trapped, worthless, alone, and lonely as some examples.

4. Now draw a path out to the right-hand side of the page. At the top of the path put a heading—how to reclaim the brain and create new patterns. Now ask your client and brainstorm with them: Can you list actions you take that help create new thought patterns /neural pathways and reduce the impact of the old ones? The client may mention identify my feelings. The client may also state ways of releasing feelings by tapping, movement, talking openly to a trusted friend, writing a letter to release the hurt from someone that impacted you negatively. Self-care activities such as

yoga, hiking, time in nature, and other self-soothing activities are mentioned as well.

5. Now do a feedback loop for behaviors that feedback to the embodied emotion, triggered thoughts and core beliefs, and ask the client: What do you do that triggers embodied emotion and increases the likelihood you will believe the thoughts and core beliefs you are wanting to distance from?

6. Drawing a triangle from the eyes out to the open page representing a vision—asking the client: Where would you like to be heading in life, what passions and interests will help motivate you to develop new neural pathways?

Ant's View versus Bird's-Eye View

This visual can be helpful for a client to get perspective on their situation. It also highlights the power of choice, particularly when one feels stuck and immobilized. To begin draw a body; in front of the body put all of the clients' present struggles, each of them encapsulated in a boxed square in front of the body.

Some questions to use to fill in the image are:

1. When you look at all these demands what is the impact on your heart? Draw a heart on the image and list all the feelings that come up. They could include anger, self-pity shame, guilt, victimization, hurt, misunderstood, fearful, despair, regret, undermined, manipulated, powerless, panic, and helpless as some examples.

2. Draw an ant near the feet of the body you have drawn. Put eyes on the ant and fill in a long triangle from the eyes of the ant to the problems and name it "the ants view." Brainstorm with your client when you are looking at your problems from ant's perspective what do you see? What thoughts do you have and do any beliefs come up around when dealing with these issues? The ant's view may include I'll never recover, this is more than I can handle, what do I do now, I need to perfect everything, what have I done wrong, why does this keep happening, what did I do to deserve this situation, I can't do all of this, I want to run away, I want out, and I'm a victim as some reflections. Put a spiral under the ant's feet and show the impact of this thinking is likely to include one spiraling into a vortex whereby the feelings and thoughts intensify. Also include behaviors that contribute to the ant's perspective and add those to the drawing.

3. Now put a bird at the top of the page and ask the client:
     When you are looking at these problems and your overall situation from a higher and detached perspective what are you seeing?

1.7 Ants View vs Bird's Eye View

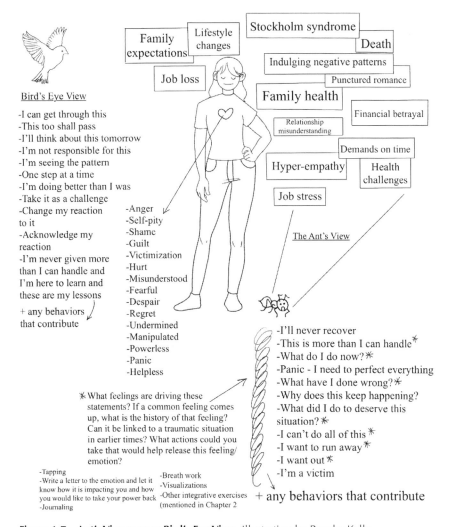

Figure 1.7   Ant's View versus Bird's-Eye View. Illustration by Brooke Kelly.

A key piece to note is that it is very challenging to imagine another perspective until the feelings, and thoughts, associated with the problems and overall situation are fully fleshed out in the drawing. A bird's perspective could include I can get through this, this too shall pass, I'll think about this tomorrow, I'm not responsible for this, I'm seeing the pattern, one step at a time, I'm doing better than I was, take it as a challenge, change my reaction to it, acknowledge my reaction, I'm never given more than I can handle and I'm here to learn and these are my lessons. Also ask the client: What behaviors help you to reach for a bird's-eye view perspective? List those in a separate category next to the list just noted.

4. Now ask the client, what are some of the strongest statements from the ant's view, put an asterisk on them. Now reflect on what feeling is driving that statement—write the feeling along with the statement. Ask the client do you feel this feeling repeatedly in your life, if so, what is the history of that emotion, link it if possible, to a traumatic situation in earlier times to understand the intensity of the repetitive thought. Now brainstorm with client what actions could you take that would help release the embodied emotion. Examples may be tapping, write a letter to the emotion and let it know how it is impacting you, and how you would like to take your power back. Regular journal writing to release, breathwork, visualizations, and other integrative exercises mentioned in chapter 2.

Impact of the Past on the Present

This drawing can be helpful to educate a client about the impact of trauma, build self-awareness in relation to how trauma manifests in everyday habits, assist the client in clearing the impact of past trauma, and develop a lifestyle that assists in moving forward. Start the visual by listing on the far left hand side of the page patterns of behavior that limit one's ability to tackle upcoming issues. They could be procrastination, perfectionism, obsessive-compulsive behavior, perseverating, over-analyzing, denial, giving over to distraction, numbing with busyness, misusing drugs, or alcohol, getting locked into a fixed routine, projecting, blaming others, co-dependency, over-involvement in others' problems as some relevant examples. On top of the patterns put 100 pounds to imply the heaviness that these behaviors produce. Next draw a body, right of the list of patterns of behavior and link the body to the past patterns with an arrow.

Some questions to use to fill in the image are:

1. Draw a triangle from the person's eyes to the open page—reflecting their lens on what happens in their life. What are some of the feelings associated with the past patterns—list them and link them to the heart and also link the heart to the list of perceptions? Now reflect on the patterns and feelings and record how it impacts the way you see future challenges. Some ideas may include situations that arise are likely out of my control, I'm being victimized by life, life's not fair, how come this keeps happening to me, when will it end, I'm never going to be able

Visual 1.8 Impact of the Past on the Present

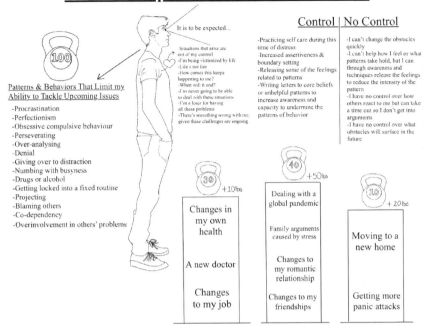

Figure 1.8   **Impact of the Past on the Present**. Illustration by Brooke Kelly.

to deal with these situations, I'm a loser for having all these problems, there's something wrong with me given these challenges are ongoing.

2. Now list a series of obstacles in front of the person. They could be in three different tall boxes—with each box list the set of problems and challenges that are creating obstacles and put a weight on each one; for instance, one box is 40 pounds of weight, another 30, and a third one 10 pounds. Ask your client "What set of obstacles are ahead of you, list a pressing problem in your life and all the interrelated issues with that problem?" For instance, one box could be the impact of recent changes. The changes could include changes in health, change in family arguments related to stress, it could be changes related to the outside world like a pandemic and all the changes it brings. Sort each set of problems into the boxes giving an appropriate weight with how much they are weighing you down.

3. Ask the client: When you look at the impact of past patterns of behavior for example procrastination, perfectionism, and obsessive-compulsive behavior ask how it influences your lens with which you view problems—how much heavier is each box given those factors? Ask the client how much that adds to each box and add that on.

4. At the top of the page add two columns—one has the heading of control, the other no control. Now ask the client: When you look at the current situation and your desire to move through obstacles what are all the factors "in your control" and all the factors "outside of your control"? The list for "in control" could include practicing self-care during this time of distress. Other examples could be increased assertiveness and boundary setting, releasing some of the feelings related to patterns, writing letters to core beliefs or unhelpful patterns to increase awareness and undermine the patterns of behavior. Whenever a pattern has a strong hold reflecting on the feeling that may be driving the pattern and releasing it with an integrative technique. Regarding "out of control" a list could be I can't change the obstacles quickly, I can't help how I feel or what patterns take hold, but I can through awareness and techniques release the feelings to reduce the intensity of the pattern. I have no control over how others react to me but can take a time out so I don't get into arguments. I have no control regarding what obstacles will surface in the future. These lists can assist the client in focusing their energy where it is likely to make the most difference, offering some empowerment when they are perhaps feeling defeated and overwhelmed.

Detaching from the Vortex of Chaos

This visual or tool is helpful for clients who find themselves in a repeated pattern of creating chaos and perceive it is as a cyclical pattern in their lives. Moving into chaos can be a coping strategy, like distraction, as it can divert attention from feelings and experiences that are perceived as overwhelming, and best avoided. Draw a maze of circles representing the vortex, name it by putting above it "vortex of chaos."

Some questions to use to fill in the image are:

1. What experiences keeps you in the vortex? Some responses may be fear of not being able to deal with chaos, can't do the things I used to, nobody cares, not meeting others' expectations, I'm a loser, fear of feeling feelings, fear of feeling alone, fear of failure, dealing with others, self-judgment, conforming to others and unexpected events. Then ask the client: What actions keep you locked into the vortex? Examples include getting overly involved with others' problems, doing what I don't want to do, not listening to intuition, TV taking over, doing without thinking, eating junk food, isolating, not getting dressed, and not getting out of the house.
2. Put a stick figure in the vortex and put a heart on the figure. Now with an arrow onto the open page list all the feelings one feels in the vortex,

Visual 1.9 Detaching From the Vortex of Chaos

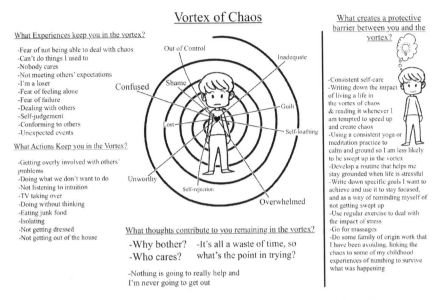

Vortex of Chaos

What Experiences keep you in the vortex?

-Fear of not being able to deal with chaos
-Can't do things I used to
-Nobody cares
-Not meeting others' expectations
-I'm a loser
-Fear of feeling alone
-Fear of failure
-Dealing with others
-Self-judgement
-Conforming to others
-Unexpected events

What Actions Keep you in the Vortex?

-Getting overly involved with others' problems
-Doing what we don't want to do
-Not listening to intuition
-TV taking over
-Doing without thinking
-Eating junk food
-Isolating
-Not getting dressed
-Not getting out of the house

Out of Control
Inadequate
Shame
Confused
Guilt
Lost
Self-loathing
Unworthy
Self-rejection
Overwhelmed

What thoughts contribute to you remaining in the vortex?

-Why bother?   -It's all a waste of time, so
-Who cares?   what's the point in trying?

-Nothing is going to really help and I'm never going to get out

What creates a protective barrier between you and the vortex?

-Consistent self-care
-Writing down the impact of living a life in the vortex of chaos & reading it whenever I am tempted to speed up and create chaos
-Using a consistent yoga or meditation practice to calm and ground so I am less likely to be swept up in the vortex
-Develop a routine that helps me stay grounded when life is stressful
-Write down specific goals I want to achieve and use it to stay focused, and as a way of reminding myself of not getting swept up
-Use regular exercise to deal with the impact of stress
-Go for massages
-Do some family of origin work that I have been avoiding, linking the chaos to some of my childhood experiences of numbing to survive what was happening

Figure 1.9   Detaching from the Vortex of Chaos. Illustration by Brooke Kelly.

linking them to the heart. The client may mention unworthy, guilt, shame, self-loathing, lost, confused, inadequate, overwhelmed, out of control, and self-rejection.

3. Next question can be: "What thoughts contribute to you remaining in the vortex?" Put the thoughts in a cloud over the head; some of the thoughts could be: Why bother? Who cares? It's all a waste of time, What's the point in trying? Nothing is going to help, and I'm never going to get out.

4. On the far-right-hand side draw a figure and put a barrier between the vortex and the figure. Now ask the client, "If you are wanting out of the vortex what are some ideas that will help propel you out, keeping in mind the vortex also has some pull over you given it helps you avoid to some degree"? Another way of putting it could be: What creates a protective barrier between you and the vortex? The client may mention consistent self-care, writing down the impact of living a life in the vortex of chaos and reading it whenever I am tempted to speed up and create chaos. Using a consistent yoga or meditation practice to calm and ground so I am less likely to be swept up in the vortex. Develop a routine that helps me stay grounded when life is stressful. Write down specific goals I want to achieve and use it to stay focused, and as a reminder to not get swept up in the chaos. Use regular exercise to deal with the impact of stress, go

for massages and do some family of origin work that I have been avoiding, linking the chaos to some of my childhood experiences of numbing to survive what was happening.

Shrinking Heart versus Expanding Heart

This visual can be helpful in times of activation of trauma, as the symptoms of hypoarousal can mimic a shrinking heart. For instance, with hypoarousal the client can show disconnection from self and others, narrow focus of attention, flat affect, shutting down, disassociation, exhaustion, numb, and memory loss. Draw two bodies representing the client, one on the far left and the other far right. Now add a shrunken heart on the body to the left and an expansive heart represented by a number of lines around the heart on the body to the right. The drawing will capture where the client is at right now, if in hypoarousal the key piece is to work with the client and ascertain if they are able to make tiny steps to move back into their window of tolerance. A first step may be attuning to the room they are in.

Visual 1.10 Shrinking Heart Versus Expanding Heart

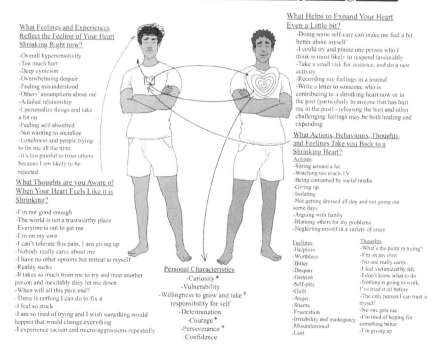

Figure 1.10   Shrinking Heart versus Expanding Heart. Illustration by Brooke Kelly.

Some questions to use to fill in the image are:

1. Ask the client what feelings and experiences reflect a feeling of their heart shrinking right now? If the client is able to verbalize then some answers might be overall hypersensitivity, too much hurt, deep cynicism, overwhelming despair, feeling misunderstood, others assumptions about me, a failed relationship, I personalize things and take a lot on, feeling self-absorbed, not wanting to socialize, loneliness and people trying to fix me all the time, it's too painful to trust others because I am likely to be rejected. If the client is finding it difficult to talk, listing the symptoms of hypoarousal they are experiencing right now and adding them to the visual may be helpful in drawing them out.

2. If the client can verbalize a little bit, enquire: What thoughts are you aware of when your heart feels like it is shrinking? Some thoughts that may be relevant are, I'm not good enough, the world is not a trustworthy place, everyone is out to get me, I'm on my own, I can't tolerate this pain, I am giving up, nobody really cares about me, I have no other options but retreat to myself, reality sucks, it takes so much from me to try and trust another person and inevitably they let me down, when will all this pain end, there is nothing I can do to fix it, I feel so stuck, I am so tired of trying, and I wish something would happen that would change everything and I experience racism and micro-aggressions repeatedly. If the client is in a pronounced hypoarousal state it may be helpful to intuit some thoughts and enquire whether they relate to the thoughts you are sharing, if they do fill them in the drawing.

3. The next step is to draw an arrow from the shrunken heart to the more expanded heart and brainstorm with the client: What helps to expand your heart even a little bit? The client may say, doing some self-care can make me feel a bit better about myself, I could try and phone one person who I think is most likely to respond favorably, take a small risk for instance, and do a new activity. Other ideas may be recording my feelings in a journal, write a letter to someone who is contributing to a shrinking heart now or in the past, particularly to anyone that has hurt one in the past, releasing the hurt and other challenging feelings may be both healing and expanding. If the client feels cynicism or bitterness at times, it may be an area to explore regarding "what experiences led to the cynicism and bitterness and is the client willing to explore them and add them to the drawing."

4. Now draw an arrow from the expanded heart back to the shrinking heart and ask the client: What actions, behaviors, thoughts, and feelings take you back to a shrinking heart? The client may talk about sitting around a lot, watching too much TV, being consumed by social media, giving up, isolating, not getting dressed all day and not going out some days, arguing with family, blaming others for my problems, neglecting myself in a

variety of areas. The feelings may be helpless, worthless, bitter, despair, distrust, self-pity, guilt, shame, anger, frustration, irritability, inadequate, misunderstood, and lost as some examples. Thoughts that may result are what's the point in trying, no one really cares, I'm on my own, I feel victimized by life, I don't know what to do, nothing is going to work I've tried it all before, the only person I can trust is myself, no one gets me, I'm tired of hoping for something better and I'm giving up.

5. Now put another arrow from the heart to a different part of the open page and add a heading "personal characteristics." Lastly one can brainstorm with your client: What personal characteristics help in the heart expansion process? The list could include curiosity, vulnerability, willingness to grow, take responsibility for self, determination, courage, perseverance, and confidence. Ask the client to put an asterisk next to any characteristic that they think they can own, even a little bit.

Building Strength in Times of Suffering

This visual can assist clients when victimization or self-pity gets triggered during a time of suffering. It can be helpful for the client to be aware of choices that they do have despite the situation. Start the visual by putting a stick figure on the far left hand side of the page with a line under them reflecting a road or path. Now indicate that the path drops off into a huge pit and put the figure falling into the pit, calling it broken places.

Some questions to use to fill in the image are:

1. What are some of the events that led you to fall into the pit? The client might add Christmas, procrastination, workplace stresses, car accident, disappointments, feeling invalidated, financial pressures, health issues, and conflict as some examples.

2. Now put circles, around the head of the image falling into the pit, to reflect thoughts that are contributing to falling in. The thoughts may be, here we go again, nothing ever works out, I can't cope with everyday challenges, why bother, it's all too much, this always happens to me, there is nothing I can do, it's as if I am getting punished for just trying in life, I give up and there is no point in trying to get to a better place.

3. Next step is to put a heart on the figure falling into the pit. Put an arrow from the heart to the open page and list all the feelings the client is feeling when they experience suffering taking over. The feelings might be hopeless, alone, out of control, despair, blah, depressed, agitated, isolated, desperate, panicked, ungrateful, victimized, and angry.

4. The next question to ask the client is: Whether they feel ready to work at getting out of the pit or whether the task feels too monumental right

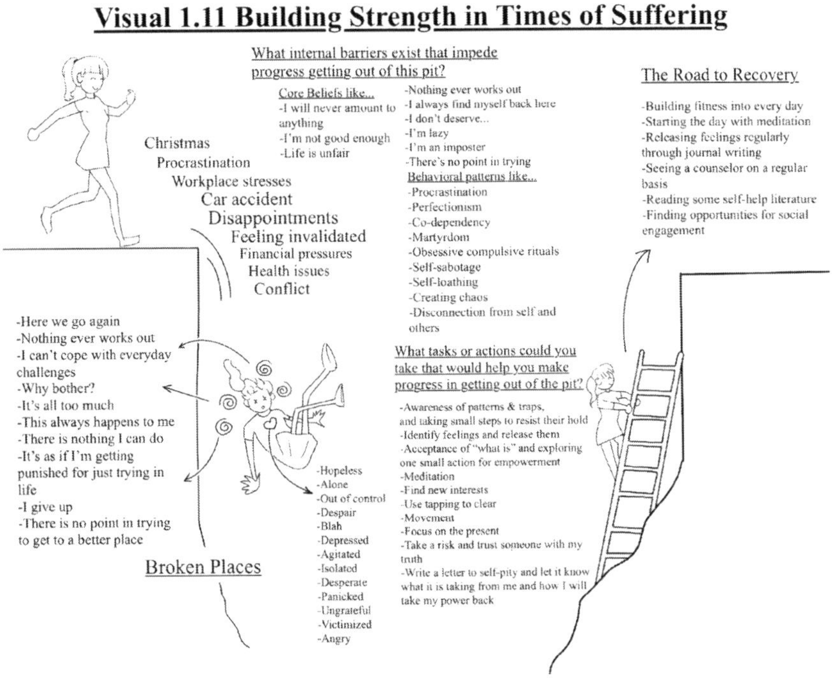

Visual 1.11 Building Strength in Times of Suffering

What internal barriers exist that impede progress getting out of this pit?

Core Beliefs like...
-I will never amount to anything
-I'm not good enough
-Life is unfair
-Nothing ever works out
-I always find myself back here
-I don't deserve...
-I'm lazy
-I'm an imposter
-There's no point in trying

Behavioral patterns like...
-Procrastination
-Perfectionism
-Co-dependency
-Martyrdom
-Obsessive compulsive rituals
-Self-sabotage
-Self-loathing
-Creating chaos
-Disconnection from self and others

Christmas
Procrastination
Workplace stresses
Car accident
Disappointments
Feeling invalidated
Financial pressures
Health issues
Conflict

The Road to Recovery

-Building fitness into every day
-Starting the day with meditation
-Releasing feelings regularly through journal writing
-Seeing a counselor on a regular basis
-Reading some self-help literature
-Finding opportunities for social engagement

-Here we go again
-Nothing ever works out
-I can't cope with everyday challenges
-Why bother?
-It's all too much
-This always happens to me
-There is nothing I can do
-It's as if I'm getting punished for just trying in life
-I give up
-There is no point in trying to get to a better place

Broken Places

What tasks or actions could you take that would help you make progress in getting out of the pit?

-Awareness of patterns & traps, and taking small steps to resist their hold
-Identify feelings and release them
-Acceptance of "what is" and exploring one small action for empowerment
-Meditation
-Find new interests
-Use tapping to clear
-Movement
-Focus on the present
-Take a risk and trust someone with my truth
-Write a letter to self-pity and let it know what it is taking from me and how I will take my power back

-Hopeless
-Alone
-Out of control
-Despair
-Blah
-Depressed
-Agitated
-Isolated
-Desperate
-Panicked
-Ungrateful
-Victimized
-Angry

Figure 1.11   **Building Strength in Times of Suffering**. Illustration by Brooke Kelly.

now? A critical piece to process with the client is the importance of timing. It can be helpful for the client to understand, from a trauma-informed perspective, that the feelings we are feeling right now can have a link back to childhood trauma, so it may not be easy to make progress. Alerting the client to internal barriers that may also impede progress is critical, this helps to foster self-compassion and patience. Some barriers are internalized core beliefs, formed in times of trauma. Some examples are I will never amount to anything, I'm not good enough, life is unfair, nothing ever works out, I always find myself back here, I don't deserve . . . , I'm lazy, I'm an imposter and there's no point in trying. Other internal barriers could be patterns of behavior that contribute to being stuck, for example, procrastination, perfectionism, co-dependency, martyrdom, obsessive-compulsive rituals, self-sabotage, self-loathing, creating chaos, and disconnection from self and others. Acknowledging internal barriers, naming them, and exploring ways to undermine their hold is an important piece of the work going forward, and can help to create the momentum for change.

5. If the client is ready to start putting one foot in front of the other to start climbing out of the pit, draw a figure on a ladder on the far-right-hand

side of the pit. The rungs of the ladder could represent different steps in the process. Next ask the client: What tasks or action will help you make progress in getting out of the pit? The client might mention, awareness of patterns and traps and take small steps to resist their hold, identify feelings and release them, acceptance of "what is" and explore what is one small action for empowerment. Some examples for empowerment could be meditation, find new interests, use tapping to clear, movement, focus on the present, take a risk and trust someone with my truth and write a letter to self-pity and let it know what it is taking from me and how I will take my power back.

6. Draw a line from the top of the pit out to the far right and call it road of recovery. Now list some long-term lifestyle habits that one could incorporate over time to assist in bypassing another pitfall in the future. These might include building fitness into every day, starting the day with meditation, releasing feelings regularly through journal writing, seeing a counselor on a regular basis, reading some self-help literature, and finding opportunities for social engagement as some examples of lifestyle changes.

Dealing with Others' Issues and Judgment's Role

This visual can be applicable to clients struggling with "others" issues and judging self as a consequence. Often dealing with others emotional issues can stir up a range of feelings, and self-judgment can be a response to feelings of inadequacy, helplessness, fear, and guilt. Start the image by drawing the client on the far-right corner of the page facing another person who has a backpack of problems. Each stone in the backpack is a problem in their life that they are experiencing; it could include conflict with another, someone else's avoidance, their physical pain, their lack of purpose, depression, anxiety, addictions, their difficulty maintaining work, a long-term struggle with trauma, suicidality, mental illness, or resistance to seeking help.

Some questions to use to fill in the image are:

1. Draw a heart on the figure representing the client, list all the feelings that another person's problems trigger. For instance, it could include despair, devastated, fear, frustration, empty, inadequate, helplessness, victimization, hopeless, trapped, stifled, controlled, isolated, discouraged, out of control, guilt, and shame as some examples.
2. Now put circles around the head to indicate the judgments that are directed to self and others, that are triggered by the situation of the other persons concerns. They could be I don't know what to do, why can't they just fix the problem, I am not strong enough to deal with this, I never say

Visual 1.12 Dealing With Others' Issues and Judgement's Role

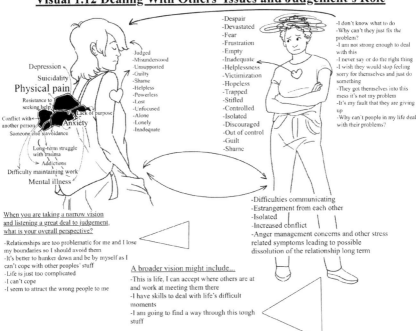

Figure 1.12   Dealing with Others Issues and Judgments Role. Illustration by Brooke Kelly.

or do the right thing, I wish they would stop feeling sorry for themselves and just do something, they got themselves into this mess it's not my problem, it's my fault that they are giving up, and why can't people in my life deal with their problems.

3. Now put a heart on the "other" person with a backpack. What might they be feeling in reaction to the judgment or reaction from their family member or friend? A list of feelings could be judged, misunderstood, unsupported, guilty, shame, helpless, powerless, lost, unfocused, alone, lonely, and inadequate.

4. Now draw an arrow linking the two figures and list the consequence of the present dynamic. It could include difficulties communicating, estrangement from each other, isolated, increased conflict, anger management concerns, and other stress-related symptoms leading to possible dissolution of the relationship in the long term.

5. Now show two differing set of responses. From the eyes of the left-hand figure show a narrow vision and a wide range vision. Ask the client: When you are taking a narrow vision and listening a great deal to

judgment what is your overall perspective? It might be relationships are too problematic for me and I lose my boundaries so I should avoid them, it's better to hunker down and be by myself as I can't cope with other people's stuff, life is just too complicated, and I can't cope, and I seem to attract the wrong people to me. A broader vision may include this is life, I can accept where others are at and work at meeting them there, I have skills to deal with life's difficult moments, and I am going to find a way through this tough stuff.

Resisting Mainstream Cultural Values—Finding an Alternative Paradigm

This visual is powerful for clients critiquing aspects of a society that are structurally undermining, unsafe, challenging, or abhorrent to them and that are still reminiscent of colonial structures and values that are slow in changing at the present time, despite pressures from social justice movements. Their alienation may be due to colonial practices, eurocentrism, racism, ableism, homophobia, misogyny, patriarchal structures, transphobia, excessive

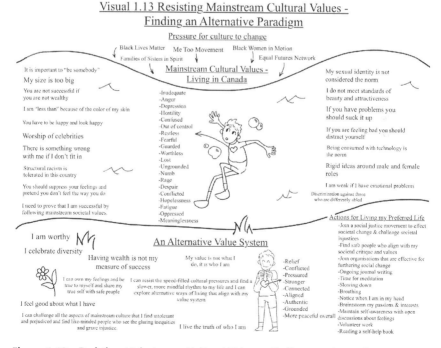

Figure 1.13 Resisting Mainstream Cultural Values—Finding an Alternative Paradigm. Illustration by Brooke Kelly.

materialism, idolization of youth and beauty, and class discrimination to name a few. This visual can assist in bolstering against re-victimization and resisting mainstream cultural pressures. Start the visual by drawing a wide river and title the river mainstream cultural values—living in Canada.

   Some questions to use to fill in the image are:

1. What are some of the mainstream cultural values in this society that you are not in agreement with, and cause some despair, alienation, tension, rage, or other feelings within you? Write down your client's response in the mainstream cultural river. Some examples named could be you are not successful if you are not wealthy, you should suppress your feelings and pretend you don't feel the way you do, worship of celebrities, rigid ideas around male and female roles, there is something wrong with me if I don't fit in, structural racism is tolerated in this country, that my sexual identity is not considered the norm, that I do not meet standards of beauty and attractiveness, that my size is too big, that I am "less than" because of the color of my skin, that if you are feeling bad you should distract yourself, that I am weak if I have emotional problems, if you have problems you should suck it up, you have to be happy and look happy, that being consumed with technology is the norm, that I need to prove that I am successful by following mainstream societal values and it is important to "be somebody" as some examples. Draw the client's body in the river and put a heart on it. Now brainstorm with the client the feelings they feel while being swept away in the mainstream cultural river. They may include inadequate, anger, depression, rage, rejected, hostility, confused, out of control, restless, fearful, guarded, worthless, lost, ungrounded, numb, despair, conflicted, hopelessness, fatigue, meaninglessness, and oppressed to name a few. Add in some cultural movements at the top of the river with arrows pointing down that are putting pressure on mainstream societal values to change. They could include, Black Lives Matter, Me Too, Families of Sisters in Spirit, Black Women in Motion, and Equal Futures Network as some examples.

2. Now draw a bank alongside the river and name the bank "an alternative value system" Ask the client: What are some of the values you would like to live by which undermine and contradict mainstream values you find abhorrent, unsafe, and/or abusive? Put in the answers in the bank running alongside the river. Some of the responses may include, I celebrate diversity, I feel good about what I have, I live the truth of who I am, having wealth is not my measure of success, I can own my feelings and be true to myself and share my true self with safe people, I am worthy, I can challenge all the aspects of mainstream culture that I find intolerant and

prejudiced and find like-minded people who see the glaring inequities and grave injustice, my value is not what I do it is who I am, I can resist the speed filled cultural pressures and find a slower, more mindful rhythm to my life and I can explore alternative ways of living that align with my value system. Now draw the client again with a heart and enquire what feelings are generated when the client is following their alternative value system. The feelings may include pressured, conflicted, stronger, connected, aligned, authentic, relief, grounded, and more peaceful overall.

3. Now with an arrow directed from the bank of the river to the open page ask the client to make a list of "actions for living my preferred life." It could include join a social justice movement to challenge societal norms and injustices, find safe people who align with one's own societal critique, ongoing journal writing, time for meditation, slowing down, join organizations that are accelerating social change, breathing, notice when I am in my head, brainstorm my passions and interests, maintain self-awareness with open discussions about feelings, volunteer work, and reading a self-help book as some examples.

Old You and New Emerging You

This visual can be very helpful when a client has made some significant changes; it assists with validation and motivation to continue the change process. The visual can assist the client in being clear about, what shifts they have been able to make, what habits or lifestyle issues undermined their progress, and how their old way of being was impacting their everyday experience. To start the process, draw two bodies on either side of the page leaving space on either side each body to fill in text. Title the body on the left as the "old you" and the one on the right as the "new and emerging you." Now start with the "old you."

Some questions to use to fill in the image are:

1. Ask the client to describe some characteristics of their "old self" including feelings and behaviors. Some examples may include follows societal rules, avoidance, numb, distracted, self-denial, tense, insecure, disconnected, needy, shame, self-judgment, I'm inadequate, I'm broken, I'm unworthy, I'm not good enough, It's not fair, self-pity, I give up, I'm a victim, I'm never going to change, I don't want to . . , I hate. . , no reason to get up, I'm in a slump, pretending, not trusting, no faith, isolated, obsess, lonely, erase ourselves, no joy, limited, repetitive, stuck in a cycle, always an excuse, work excessively, lose myself, no one understands, no one wants to see the real me, cynical and bitter, and I'm jealous of others. Now add bricks under the feet of the old you and list

Visual 1.14 Old You and New Emerging You

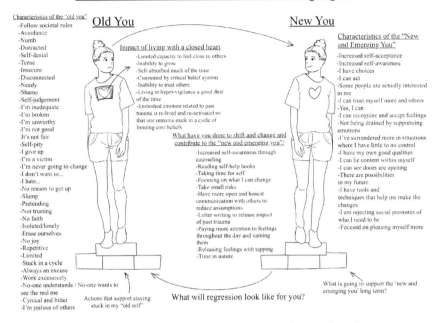

Figure 1.14   Old You and New Emerging You. Illustration by Brooke Kelly.

those actions that support one staying stuck in ones "old self." It could be, countless hours of social media, sleeping and eating excessively, smoking weed every day, and withdrawing socially.

2. Draw a heart on the body and put various lines around it as if the heart is trapped in walls, put an arrow from the heart and ask the client: When the old you dominates what is the impact of living with a closed heart? The client may mention, limited capacity to feel close to others, inability to grow, self-absorbed much of the time, consumed by a critical belief system, inability to trust others, living in hypervigilance a good deal of the time, clinician could add if client agrees embodied emotion related to past trauma is re-lived and reactivated, and remain stuck in a cycle of limiting core beliefs.

3. Now put an arrow from the body of the "old you" to the "new and emerging you" body. Ask the client what have they done to shift and change and contribute to the "new and emerging you." The client could mention increased self-awareness through counseling, reading self-help books, taking time for self, focusing on what I can change, take small risks, have more open and honest communication with others to reduce assumptions, letter writing to release the impact of past trauma, paying more attention

to feelings throughout the day and naming them, releasing feelings with tapping and time in nature.

4. Now enquiring re "What are the characteristics of the 'new and emerging you'?" The client may mention, increased self-acceptance, increased awareness, I have choices, I can act, some people are actually interested in me, I can trust myself more and others, yes I can, I can recognize and accept feelings, not being drained by suppressing emotions, I've surrendered more in situations where I have little to no control, I have my own good qualities, I can be content within myself, I can see doors are opening, there are more possibilities in my future, I have tools and techniques that help me make changes and I am rejecting societal pressures of who I need to be, and focused on pleasing myself more.

5. Now put some bricks under the feet of the new and emerging you and brainstorm with the client "What is going to support the new and emerging you long term?" Some of the answers may be in the list of what contributed to the change but there may be some other actions that would be helpful to integrate long term, perhaps for embodied emotion increased attention to body work, developing a wider range of interests, and establishing clearer boundaries with those who do not see ones change for example.

6. Also add to the drawing a feedback loop from the new and emerging you to the old you and back again to symbolize that regression is often to be expected. Ask the client "What will regression look like to you?" Add these ideas under the feedback loop arrows.

Betrayal

This visual may be helpful for those clients who have experienced betrayal in an intimate relationship, or betrayal of a friend or work colleague. It can also include self-betrayal where one has dishonored one's own integrity for a short-term gain, or a betrayal of deeply held convictions or values. The betrayal in the drawing will focus on the betrayal of an intimate relationship. To start the process, draw two figures facing one another, the figure on the left has a jagged line splitting the two sides of the heart, the other figure also has a heart on the figure, but it has walls around it.

Some questions to use to fill in the image are:

1. Now draw arrows from the figure who betrayed the other person and describe what constituted the betrayal? It could be, having an affair, being perceived as taking advantage of the person in some way, betraying an agreement and demanding more money, using the person for personal or financial gain, not being honest or up front with intentions and taking

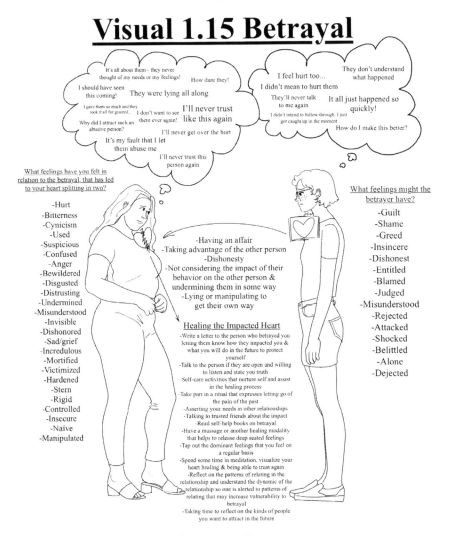

Figure 1.15   Betrayal. Illustration by Brooke Kelly.

advantage of trust, being disloyal and talking about the person to others, not considering the impact of their behavior on the person and undermining them in some way, lying or manipulating to get their own way and dishonoring their generosity.

2. Now ask the client "What feelings have you felt in relation to the betrayal, that has led to your heart feeling split in two?" It could include hurt, bitterness, cynicism, used, suspicious, confused, enraged, anger, stupefied, bewildered, disgusted, distrusting, undermined, misunderstood, unseen,

invisible, dishonored, incredulous, sad, grief, lost, mortified, victimized, hardened, stern, rigid, controlled, insecure, naïve, and manipulated to name a few.

3. Now draw a large bubble over the head of this figure and ask the client what thoughts are triggered by the betrayal? Some thoughts maybe, I should have seen this coming, why did I allow myself to be manipulated, how dare they, who do they think they are trying to get away with it, I'll never trust this person again, how abusive, what sort of a person are they, they were lying all along, what did I do to attract such an abusive person, it's all about them, they never thought of my needs or my feelings, who else shouldn't I be trusting, I gave them so much and they took it all for granted, it's my fault that I let them abuse me, I'll never trust like this again, I'll never get over the hurt, and I don't want to see them ever again.

4. Now the focus moves to the person who betrayed. Brainstorm with the client feelings they may be feeling it may be, guilt, shame, greed, insincere, dishonest, entitled, blamed, judged, misunderstood, rejected, attacked, shocked, belittled, alone, lonely, and dejected. Thoughts they may be having, captured in a bubble over their head could be, I didn't mean to hurt them, they don't understand what happened, it all just happened so quickly, I didn't intend to follow through I just got caught up in the moment, they'll never talk to me again, I feel hurt too and how do I make this better?

5. Lastly put an arrow from the heart to an open page and put a title "healing the impacted heart." Brainstorm with the client all the actions they can take that will help them heal from the betrayal. It could include, write a letter to the person who betrayed you letting them know how they impacted you, and what you will do in the future to protect yourself, talk to the person if they are open and willing to listen and state your truth, self-care activities that nurture self and assist in the healing process, take part in a ritual that expresses letting go of the pain of the past, asserting your needs in other relationships, talking to trusted friends about the impact, read self-help books on betrayal, have a massage or another healing modality that helps to release deep seated feelings, tap out the dominant feelings that you feel on a regular basis, spend some time in meditation, visualize your heart healing and being able to trust again, visualize those people in your life who you can trust, seek to understand the dynamic of the relationship so one is alerted to patterns of relating that may increase vulnerability to betrayal in the future, and taking time to reflect on what are the characteristics of people you want to attract in the future.

Feeling Unlovable

The description and questions to ask on this image are on page

Visual 1.16 Feeling Unlovable

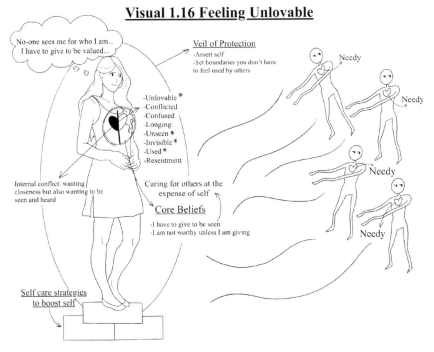

Figure 1.16   **Feeling Unlovable**. Illustration by Brooke Kelly.

Experiential Unity Model and Format for Group Therapy Sessions

Steps—Experiential Unity Model and Group Work

Step 1—Breathing/mindfulness/visualization/body scan for example to calm and ground.

Step 2—Breathe and feel—identify where tension/sensation/urges are held in the body, breathe into this area, and see if a feeling can be identified. Clients go around the circle and state a feeling in one or two words (no explanation needed).

Step 3—Check in—Check in can vary. Crisis stabilization group, for instance; Highlights and challenges of the week and how did you do on your action plan?

Other groups—emphasize the visual the week before, for instance, tool on slowing down—Did you slow down or speed up this last week and how did you do on your action plan?

Other check in is related to overall group theme—for example, a self-compassion group—check in could be "Did you mainly judge and criticize yourself this last week or did you take time to reflect on ways to build self-compassion and how did you do on your action plan?"

Each client after the check in process receives brief feedback on strengths from one group member and one facilitator. The client does not comment on the feedback, rather takes time to reflect on it and then accept or reject it internally.

Step 4—A tentative theme proposed to the group—group feedback on theme, could just be nodding heads. Once there is agreement re the theme a visual is drawn on the board that captures the overriding theme of the group. Fill in all aspects of the visual to capture experiences from clients in the group, paying particular attention to their present struggles, embodied emotion, and in the last segment focus on what will help to alleviate the struggle.

Step 5—Shaking for a couple of minutes and Kundalini yoga moves to release tension in the body (see list of Kundalini exercise on page 39–40).

Step 6—Wrap up—What stood out in the group today and what is an action plan for the week.

Expanded versions for each step in the group work process are as follows.

Step 1—This step is similar to the start of an individual therapy session. The mindfulness component can include breathwork, mindfulness, visualizations, tapping, movement, body scan, qigong, stretching, or any other relaxation technique that assists the client in connecting with their body. If the clients are willing and able, I have also tried putting on calming music and have given each client a hard ball to use on areas of their body that feel stiff. Clients have pressed against a wall, positioning the ball in a particular position, or have sat on the hard ball, and practiced deep breathing as a way of releasing tension and/or embodied emotion in the body. For clients who are not comfortable with this exercise they can go for a brief mindful walk.

Step 2—Breathe and feel. Once the relaxation component is over asking clients to close their eyes if they are comfortable, or keep their eyes fixed on the floor, and then the facilitator states we are now going to breathe and feel. One could add "using your breath like a fishing line to retrieve feelings in your body." For clients who are uncomfortable "feeling," they can bypass this process and state the feeling they do feel in the round, for instance, it may be numb, empty, or disconnected.

The facilitator now asks "Who is ready to state one or two feeling words?" A client may say sad, then it moves onto the next person in the circle until everyone has gone. This process assists the clients to move out of their heads and into their feeling state. It is a primer for the latter part of the group whereby clients are able to state some of the feelings they feel for the visual.

Step 3—Check in. Even though the "check in" is varied according to the group, clients are reminded to in all groups to include as many articulated feelings as possible in the content of their "check-in." In a crisis stabilization group, the check in that seemed to work best is, "What are the highlights and challenges of your week, and how did you do on your action plan?" This check in engages the client in a process of releasing their present overriding concerns while also talking about highlights. This process of remembering both a challenge and highlight at the same time assists in the process of reconditioning. Linda Graham in *Bouncing Back* states,

> the key to reconditioning is holding any two contradictory experiences or memories in awareness at the same time, a state known as simultaneous dual awareness, and to intensify the focus on the positive memory while also remaining aware of the negative memory we have chosen to rewire. This simultaneous awareness requires practice. If it is challenging at first, you can begin by switching back and forth between the two memories, always refreshing and strengthening the positive memory so that it becomes stronger. Eventually there can be a simultaneous awareness of the two memories. This creates the simultaneous neural firing that allows the two memories to reconsolidate together in a new network. (Graham, 2013, p. 121)

Another "check in" that can be helpful to coalesce the different group sessions together is for clients to report on the prior week's visual image. For instance, if the theme the week before was about anger management, then a check in question a week later could be "Did you mainly manage your anger this last week or did it manage you, and how did you do on your action plan?" Another example with an eight-session self-compassion group, a "check in" could be "In this last week was self-compassion weaker or stronger than self-criticism and self-judgment?" In a stress management group, anxiety management group, depression management group, and an eating disorder group I have used the stress/pain container—visual 1.1 as the first image in week one of the group. My rationale is that depression, anxiety, stress, obsessive-compulsive behavior, and eating behaviors of starving or bingeing are symptoms of trauma. The stress/pain container tool emphasizes self-connection as a way of releasing past trauma. A helpful check in with the stress/pain container in week two and for the rest of the group series could be, "Did you mainly connect and heal this last week or did you find yourself running away from feelings, disconnecting, and adding to the weight of your container?" I have used this "check in" for many years in group work and have found the impact profound in teaching clients about trauma. By repeating the "check in" phrase regularly and hearing other clients responding to the phrase re connection and disconnection, clients have demonstrated learning around what helps them heal, regulate their nervous system, and also become increasingly aware of how their lifestyle impacts their capacity to connect somatically. (See chapter four on cultural traps to healing.) These concepts can have a profound impact on the shifts that clients can make in a group setting. The stress/pain container tool and the range of concepts it teaches can have a profound impact on the client's capacity to grow and change within the group setting. The stress/pain container tool is also challenging cultural messages that undermine the healing process. Some of the core beliefs I have heard from clients repeatedly in groups are: I shouldn't feel the way I do, suck it up, I am supposed to be happy, if you feel an uncomfortable feeling get busy, distract, pretend it's not there, there's something wrong with me, and I'm a loser for feeling the way I do. I have seen the result of these beliefs repeatedly in encouraging clients to disconnect from self, get lost, lose their way, and lose contact with the deepest part of themselves which is critical to the healing process. "I shouldn't feel the way I do" I believe has single-handedly made a huge impact on levels of depression, anxiety, stress, self-rejection, and self-criticism evident in multitude of clients seeking help.

After the "check in" from a client, each client remains silent while one group member and one facilitator, in that order, give feedback on strengths they noticed. Clients are reminded to stay silent so they can listen to the feedback at a deep level, and it can also assist them in processing and remembering the feedback. I noted before I introduced the component of not responding to the feedback, that clients would minimize their strengths or at times undermine the feedback. Taking the time to be silent seems to give many clients permission to receive and reflect on the feedback, and I do add accept the parts you like and reject what doesn't fit in your own mind. The impact of "feedback on strengths" process has a significant effect on the group as a whole and shifts in group members, the following are some of the benefits I have witnessed over the years:

- The "feedback on strengths" process has a significant impact on "universality" felt in the group whereby members frequently comment they no longer feel alone in their struggle.

- There is more credibility in the feedback from a peer, who is also struggling, than the group therapist, and this likely helps in the integration of the feedback overall.
- With clients practicing giving feedback on strengths, they are more likely to see strengths in others in their lives and help them attune to their own strengths.
- For both the clients and therapist to give feedback on strengths an emphasis is put on bottom-up processing, it helps to level the power differential between clinician and client.
- This process seems to have an impact on overall engagement in the group; clients are playing an active role in assisting each other, without giving advice.
- Clients having a consistent role in feedback, frees up the group facilitators momentarily, so they can step back and "see what is happening" and experience the undercurrent of the group to develop a theme for the image.

Over the years I have frequently been moved by clients' feedback. I have marveled at their capacity to see things that I don't see and to articulate it in a profoundly sensitive manner. At times there may be a long pause before a member comes forth with feedback, but in the last decade using this consistently in all groups, I cannot recall one instance where a client hasn't received any feedback at all from a group member. At times, when the client has had a really challenging week and feels consumed by their struggle and believes they are bereft of strengths, group members have noted their honesty, or their willingness to show up despite having such a difficult week, or their capacity to show courage in the face of adversity.

As mentioned earlier, the content of the check in and the underlying feelings experienced during the check in process will assist in forming the theme for the visual.

Step 4—Creating an overriding theme, developing the theme, preamble and drawing an image. Listening for the theme of the group is a skill that takes time to develop. The John Heider quote stated earlier "knowing what is happening" reflects the degree of presence that is helpful to hear the underlying themes or deeper concerns of the group members. The depth of presence John Heider is articulating is likely challenging for most of us to attain; however, the more mindful one can be of deeper processes in the group, particularly stated or unstated feelings and body language, the more will be able to glean a theme that is universal. Each member will "check in" with their concerns; however, at a deeper level are a constellation of feelings and experiences that can connect all members of the group in a helpful and an engaging way. For instance, a check in may include one member talking about worries regarding a child, another one a recent job loss, while another may check in regarding their struggle with depression or anxiety that week, and someone else may be entering an intense process with a divorce. These are all separate experiences but at times the emotion that they trigger can be very similar. Reflecting on these experiences I may feed back to the members a struggle with feeling "out of control" with one's life circumstances and how the process creates intense vulnerability and unpredictability overall.

The theme is different each week; even if it includes similar feelings, it can be constructed with a different image so that the clients experience it as unique in that moment of their process. I have noted over the years that the images often appear repetitive re feelings even though they are presented in a different way. Similar to individual counseling and Experiential Unity model in group work I have come to learn that one week's image may deal with one layer of a particular feeling, when that feeling is released, another deeper experience with that feeling can surface, and the new visual perhaps deals with a deeper layer of a similar feeling. It is uncommon for me to use the same image twice, most of the time the images are unique to that situation.

Key questions to ponder during the "check in":

- What is a theme that links all the stories related to the "check in" together and what are some feelings that are driving the theme? Some examples may be, no matter how hard I struggle nothing seems to change with an overall feeling of helplessness and despair, no one gets me with a primary feeling of being unseen and invisible, I feel stuck in my life and can't get out with a trapped feeling evident, given my situation I don't want to make the wrong choice with a feeling of conflicted, and it is too scary to feel my feelings so distracted and numb may be evident.
- What isn't being talked about but is driving the discourse at a deep level? Sensing, intuiting, and naming the feelings can be very helpful information for detecting the overall theme?
- What are you the facilitator feeling, checking in with your own body sensations and feelings? Identifying what "your sensations as a way of knowing" are telling you and is there an overall feeling you are experiencing in the moment? It may or may not be relevant.
- When the client is sharing their situation with the group are there strong feelings expressed, or unexpressed, that are similar to others in the room?
- If a theme doesn't emerge perhaps clients are feeling stuck on islands and no one is able to understand them. Noting group dynamics is also a way to pick up important information to reflect a theme in the group. If members in the group appear quite self-absorbed due to their present predicaments, I may pick up the feeling of lonely, alone, and misunderstood. An appropriate image may be drawing people on the board and each person has a bubble around them so a first question may be: What keeps them in a

bubble? Perhaps another theme in group dynamics is a lack of trust between members with the dominant feeling of distrust. An image may be putting walls around the heart so that no one can enter, the first set of questions may enquire about why the walls around the heart are necessary?

- The theme in the group may also relate to external factors such as a member of the group having a recent suicide attempt, or the impact of living through a pandemic, or it may be the last group of a well-bonded group so undisclosed grief may be apparent. A key piece is to glean what are the dominant feelings in the group, are they stated or unstated, what is the members body language telling you about what they are experiencing in the group at this moment, and intuiting and sensing a theme from what you see, hear, or sense?
- Another common theme of the group can be "it is not safe to feel" and so most members of the group may present as numb or disconnected. The stress/pain container can be very helpful for the common experience of disconnection from self. Group members can all share their lifestyle choices or nervous dysregulation survival strategies given some of them may be experiencing symptoms of hypo or hyperarousal. The stress/pain container helps clients acknowledge disconnection from self and in essence a feeling of being stuck. It also helps clients reflect on their lifestyle choices and how they are impacting the change process. If the stress/pain container doesn't fit what other image would help to express fear of feeling?

An important piece to remember when reflecting on a theme in the group is it doesn't have to be "the best theme ever" that could be imagined. It is a tentative theme; it can always be changed according to the member's input. When I put forward a theme of the group to the members my tone is intentionally tentative, I am curious as to whether they relate to it or not, often an unconscious nodding is a clue if it hits a key piece in their struggle. Member's feedback can help tweak or change the theme to represent their concerns more clearly. That said, in my own experience most themes get rubber stamped by the group, it is rare that there is a back and forth, and my guess is that there are likely several themes that would be beneficial to run with and engage a deep therapeutic process.

Preamble before Drawing

The preamble before the drawing is a key part of the process. It is a way of helping the clients invest in the image, a meaningful precursor, helping the clients open up emotionally to the drawing. Inserting silence at various points in the preamble is key, the pause allows members time to process the theme. For example, if the theme in the group is "no matter what I do I seem to find myself feeling helpless and out of control," then the preamble could be "What I hear this week in the group is that members have made a lot of effort to take charge of their lives, and effect some meaningful change, and yet no matter your efforts it feels as if something keeps pushing you back into swirling waters, where you feel helpless and out of control and I imagine also defeated—is that right—is that how people are feeling?"

Another preamble for a theme for a group of members "feeling stuck, trapped and frustrated" could be, "What I am hearing in the group today is frustration regarding your situation where you feel like you are trapped, perhaps in a box, does that fit, and you can't seem to figure a way out no matter how much you try?" Do you relate to that—what comes up for you? What are some of the other feelings besides frustration regarding being trapped in a box? Should we draw the box and start to understand your experience in the box more fully? A final example of a preamble for a theme of "feeling lost and confused" could be, "What I am hearing from the group in the check in, is that no matter how hard you try and figure things out, nothing seems to help to take away the lost and confused feeling, it is if you are hurtling through life with little or no direction, and there is uncertainty all around you—is that right—do you relate to that?"

Once clients have affirmed the preamble, or given feedback on how it should be tweaked, or what else needs to be included you are ready to reflect on what image would best represent their current feeling state. As mentioned earlier, my experience is clients are ready to engage with the image, rarely tweak or change it, and the investment process seems mellifluous.

Developing an Image

Once a theme has emerged the next step is to develop an image that fits the theme. There is no right and wrong here, and again this is a tentative process that could have some group input, however, keep in mind presenting an image is part of starting the group investment process. Therefore, it is helpful to present an image that facilitates deep therapeutic engagement and assists the clients in feeling heard and understood in their struggle. Most of the time my co-facilitator or I have come up with the image but were also open to feedback if it was offered. The image has no limits on what it can or can't be, there are no rules on developing an image, it is over to you and your co-facilitators imagination. An important piece though is that the more complexity that can be built into the drawing the more powerful it is. I try as much as possible to move away from either/or, essentially a black/white analysis of the situation. I am always striving to sit in the gray of it all. A case in point is the "old you" or "new emerging you." Although this starts out as an either/or scenario, building in regression, behaviors and actions that support both states help to muddy the waters and present an image that is in flux and open to both helpful and regressive changes as well.

Drawing an actual body, or several bodies, fits some of the tools, and then add different tangents to the body to flesh out the drawing. Some tangents could be, what are you feeling, listing feelings from the heart, any relevant thoughts, what is the body standing on, what is above the body, what is one's experience in the body overall, who is surrounding the body as a few possible explorations. However, some images are more effectively represented as metaphors, for example, salmon swimming upstream to the tide of life, living life under a mushroom perhaps representing self in a vulnerable way. Another example of a metaphor being more powerful could be a depiction of a speed filled existence that leads to disconnection and a slow, rhythmic life. This could be represented as a hare and a tortoise, rather than two figures in contrasting states of movement. Looking at some of the examples in the visual images that have been added in this text may be helpful, but also exploring your own imagination and reflecting what would be an effective metaphor for capturing the present experience of clients in the group, and an image that would also reflect their current feeling states.

Drawing the image can also be a challenge, this is one I have experienced acutely, in fact in many a group once I got up to draw the image the clients would start to laugh knowing my drawing ability was suspect at best. The clients would disagree wholeheartedly that my rabbit did not look like a rabbit or they would say emphatically that my mushroom looked more like a spaceship. This, although challenging at times and anxiety provoking, provided a unique bonding moment in that both the group facilitators and the clients are all experiencing some degree of vulnerability.

This mutual vulnerability also reinforces the bottom-up processing and hierarchical leveling in the group. A key piece as mentioned earlier in all drawings is to use different color markers for different concepts, clients have educated me many a time of how important this is. They often include in their wrap up a reference to the color of the text on the board, for instance; I am going to be more aware of when I am in the red zone and try and move to more behaviors in the green, as soon as I am conscious of regressing.

The images most often are spontaneous and drawn from "in the moment" in the group as described in the above process. There are also times when the images can be fixed and pre-prescribed because of a specific theme of a group. A further scenario could be one or two images may be fixed and the rest spontaneous. In the group therapy programs I worked at for 30 years all of the groups had a title, and clients chose the group from the title or name of the group. For instance, group names that were commonly used were: Coping with Depression group, Anxiety management group, Self-esteem group, Self-compassion group, Rapid access group, Stress Management group, and

Mindfulness and relaxation group. Most of the above-mentioned groups were run with manuals with a cognitive behavioral therapy (CBT) focus and pre-prescribed material regardless of what the clients were experiencing in the group. I co-facilitated each one of these groups and adapted Experiential Unity model to the group theme. I incorporated some of the CBT handouts that fit with the theme and intentionally did not follow the manuals given the CBT model was co-facilitated with a left brain, top-down processing orientation. Instead drew the theme from inner processes of group members experience at that time and integrated relevant CBT handout material.

Here are some examples of adaptations regarding including Experiential Unity model in themed groups, for instance, a Coping with Depression group, an Anxiety management, and an eating disorder group. I ran the first group for the Depression, Anxiety, and Eating disorder groups with the visual image of the Stress/Pain container. Each subsequent week I referred to the image with the check-in sentence "Did you mainly connect with yourself this last week and potentially drain depression/anxiety/eating disorder symptoms or did you disconnect and find you added to them?" In week two I would do a visualization where clients drew depression/anxiety or their eating disorder and then at home wrote letters to the visual image they drew.

The visualization exercise, for clients willing to take part and with a capacity to regulate their nervous system, would include the following. Clients turn their chairs around and face the outside of the circle, then close their eyes if they can, or keep their eyes fixed on the floor, and start to do some mindful breathing and relaxing. The facilitator now guides the group through a guided visualization. "You are at home, relaxing in a comfortable chair or couch with nothing to do but relax. You are aware of the sounds of birds outside and feeling the warmth of the sun come through a window, you sink deeper into the chair or couch and start to breathe more deeply. Just breathe and relax. After a while you hear a knock at the door, you are not expecting anyone, but you get up and go to the door and you decide to open it and see who is there. When you open the door, you are staring at (insert issue here for instance) depression, anxiety, or your eating disorder, what does it look like, feel like and smell like? What feelings are you feeling when you look at it? What would you like to say back to it? Now, take a deep breath, and close the door on depression/anxiety or eating disorder and then go back to your comfortable place. You start to breathe again, releasing any tension from your body whilst noting body sensation, slowly coming back to your safe place knowing depression/anxiety or eating disorder is on the other side of the door. Now before you open your eyes reflect on what you saw, what image comes to mind, how can you depict what you saw?"

Then clients are offered paper and colored pens and asked to symbolize what they saw when they opened the door. When the clients have drawn something, they are asked to give it a name, for instance, "my tormentor" or "suffocating fog". Clients, if comfortable, are asked to share their drawings with the group, explaining to the group why they drew what they did. The technique of externalizing "the problem" is a narrative therapy technique and is highly adaptable to a wide range of situations. I have found the drawings clients have shared as powerful and they seem to help inspire each other to tackle depressive, anxiety, or eating disorder symptoms in a different way. Clients are asked, as part of their action plan, to write a letter to their drawing and to read it to the group the following week if willing. The letter captures how (the tormentor, for example) has impacted your life and what has it stolen from you and how would you like to take your power back from (the tormentor).

Here are two examples of letters I wrote which captured some of the themes I have heard addressed in clients' letters:

Coping with Depression Group Letter to Suffocating Fog

Dear Suffocating Fog,

I am so completely exhausted of you and sick of you hanging around, taking up my air, sucking my energy so I can't even get out of bed in the morning. I know you now, I have known you ever since I was eleven years old when my father died. That is when you first started to visit me. You knew I was vulnerable, suffocating fog, yes you knew I was in a crisis, so you came and took the little air I had left. You always visit me in the morning, you know mornings are hard for me and that is when I struggle the most. So, you come down on me like a huge load of steel, making it hard for me to think, to see the day ahead of me. I feel so suffocated by you—all I can do at times is put the covers over my head and try and imagine you are not there. You make me frightened to get out of bed, to face the things I must do, you are evil suffocating fog, an evil draining force.

I know your wily ways, you tempt me with sleep, I can see your tricks now, the longer I sleep the more you get a hold. In fact, I see all the tricks you have been playing on me, so you get stronger, and I get weaker. You love it when I watch countless hours of television, or scroll endlessly on my cell phone, then you take over and send all the thoughts that are so painful to hear. You tell me I am useless and will never amount to anything repeatedly until I feel utterly tormented. You also dissuade me from answering the phone saying to me that I won't know what to say, and that no-one is really interested in me anyway. When I want to try new things, like go to an exercise class, you tell me there is no point in it that nothing is going to take away my depression and your presence. When I feel a tiny bit of hope you try and take over my brain, so the hope I so dearly want evaporates.

Well suffocating fog, I am serving you notice. You are getting out of my life sometime soon; it is on my terms from now on. Your rent-free days are over, you better start planning ahead soon as I will have so much protection it will be hard for you to slither in. I sold my TV; I knew you wouldn't like that, but I did it knowing I would have more free time to do something uplifting for myself. I joined a Group therapy program and already I can see how you worm into other's lives too. I am onto your sneaky ways. By the way I joined an exercise class, and you were wrong, it lifts me for hours and have started to walk too which is helping my mood. I don't know if you have noticed suffocating fog, but I answer the phone every time it rings now, and again you were wrong, people do care about me and are offering me lots of support in my battle with you and your suffocating tendencies.

So suffocating fog, be on your way, get lost, go and torment yourself for a change instead of picking on people who are trying their hardest to fight back. If you try and take over again, know I have the tools and an array of tricks to pierce through your fog and see to the other side. The space in my brain is used for uplifting thoughts now, there is no more free rent suffocating fog, get lost and good riddance.

Below is an example of a letter written to Anxiety called—letter to my tormentor.

Dear Tormentor,

Since I drew a picture of you in the group and talked about your influence with other group members, I am becoming so much more aware of how you try and torment me every day. You know it's hard for me to be around people; that my voice shakes sometimes and so do my hands, but instead of an encouraging voice saying, "go Della, you can do it," you question my every move. You tell me that people think I am weird because my voice and hands shake with anxiety. You make it difficult for me to have a conversation with anyone because you tell me before I do that, I will make a fool of myself, and so I am embarrassed and ashamed before I have even opened my mouth.

The other day when I wanted to speak to my roommates and quit hiding out in my room you told me to stay inside, do not waste my time as people don't like me so there is no point in trying. Well, you know what, Tormentor, I know about you now, ever since I spoke about you in the group and talked about my drawing. Other people in the group also have someone like you, judging them with negative commentary throughout their day and undermining their every step. Well, guess what tormentor the time has come to get you out of my life, I am so sick of being anxious all the time and the difference is now I am willing to feel the other feelings in my body and I have the courage and strength to fight back. Every week the group members remind me of strengths

I didn't think I had, and I am starting to believe them. I used to give in to you, but those days are gone tormentor, you are history, so get out of my head and go away.

You are not going to take over my confidence anymore, not even for one more day without being detected. Sure, I know you will still talk to me and say your horrible things, but from now on you should know I am not agreeing with you. I don't believe you anymore, I have more protection from you than ever before so you will be detected. Breathing is my new best friend, when I hear you, I focus on breathing, and I can feel your negative and undermining thoughts get softer and softer the longer I breathe. I am also doing yoga exercises that clear my mind, release tension in my body and it makes it easier to muffle your voice. Every week we have tools in the group that help us resolve the past, so you have less to cling onto. So, there we have it tormentor, your power has been drained, so get out of my life—good riddance and get a life and quit trying to leach life out of me.

In most of the groups I have co-facilitated I have built in letter writing to externalize the problem and facilitate an empowerment process. I have also built letters into a Men's anger management group, grief and loss group and frequently encourage them in an individual counseling process.

Six Session Deepening Self-Connection and Healing Group

This group has six fixed images, so the theme of the group is consistent with the topic of Deepening self-connection and healing. I devised and co-facilitated this group for about 10 years, at the time it was named a Mindfulness and relaxation group. The group assists clients overall in learning mindfulness and relaxation skills to deepen their self-connection and facilitate their own healing process. Over the years looking at evaluations of the group, and noting significant changes and shifts in clients, I concluded this combination of images, emphasis on clearing techniques and nervous system regulation, and feedback on strengths provide a powerful forum for change. Part of the power of the images in the group is they offer a cultural critique of societal norms that perpetuate unhelpful beliefs about lifestyle and feelings. The images contradict societal norms of speed filled living being a preferred state of living, they confront the idea of "I shouldn't feel this way," they assist clients in becoming more aware of being in the present and away from "thinking about thinking," the images highlight choice and the importance of expanding your heart by feeling feelings, instead of intellectualizing feelings. Each group consists of the following steps in Experiential Unity model:

Step 1—Breathing, mindfulness, tapping, visualization, and so on, to start the group

Step 2—Breathe and feel and name one or two feeling words after engaging the body

Step 3—Check in:

Week 1: What would you like to get out of this series of groups and what do you do to calm and soothe your body?

Week 2: Did you mainly connect with and release stress and pain from your body or did you mainly disconnect and add to your stress/pain container? I mention to clients this is not to judge ourselves but to build awareness about how our lifestyle impacts our capacity to heal.

Week 3: Did you intentionally slow down and feel more feelings this last week or did you find yourself mainly speeding up?

Week 4: Did you take time to connect with your body and acknowledge sensation/tension and feelings or did you ignore your body for the most part and go on autopilot?

Week 5: Did you spend more time in the present this last week or did you find yourself mainly in the past or future?

Week 6: In the last week were you conscious of choices you were making on the high road or low road, where did you spend most of your time?

Step 4—Visual images for group theme of Deepening self-connection and healing.

Week 1—Stress/pain container—see Figure image 1.1

Week 2—Highway vs. country roadway of living—see Figure image 2.1

Week 3—The Body talks—see Figure image 2.2

Week 4—Living in the present or the past/future—see Figure image 2.3

Week 5—The Power of choice—see Figure image 2.4

Week 6—Heart expansion or contraction—see Figure image 2.5

Step 5—For members willing to move, stand up, and turn yourself away from the circle, closing your eyes and start to shake for a couple of minutes and then facilitator role models Kundalini yoga exercises in text page 39–40. The whole movement section takes about 10 minutes to vibrant music. Those not wishing or able to take part can stretch, go for a brief mindful walk, or remain seated turning their chair around.

Step 6—Wrap up: For each group "What stood out in the group today, how are you left feeling and what is your action plan for the next week?"

The following is a list of visuals/images for group therapy. The first six images are all utilized for the Deepening self-connection and healing group. The remainder are images /visuals of themes that have emerged in group therapy sessions.

Stress/Pain Container—1.1

This visual image is used for the first session in an Anxiety management group, Coping with Depression group, Eating disorders group, Self-compassion group, Stress management group, Mindfulness, and relaxation group, and also the Deepening self-connection group. See visual 1.1

Highway versus the country road way of living.

This tool has been utilized in this series for approximately 10 years and clients have educated me repeatedly re its impact. Many clients have not reflected on the pressures of living in a society that promotes speed at both a conscious and unconscious level. Capitalist maxims like "time is money" reinforce these ideas, as do fast-food restaurants, instant gratification, and an appetite for "quick fixes to problems." It is critical to keep in mind speed filled living may also be a result of financial constraint whereby to get by one needs to juggle two or three jobs. It is critical to build this analysis into the visual and capture that group members may be driven to speed up because of necessity and challenging economic circumstances. However,

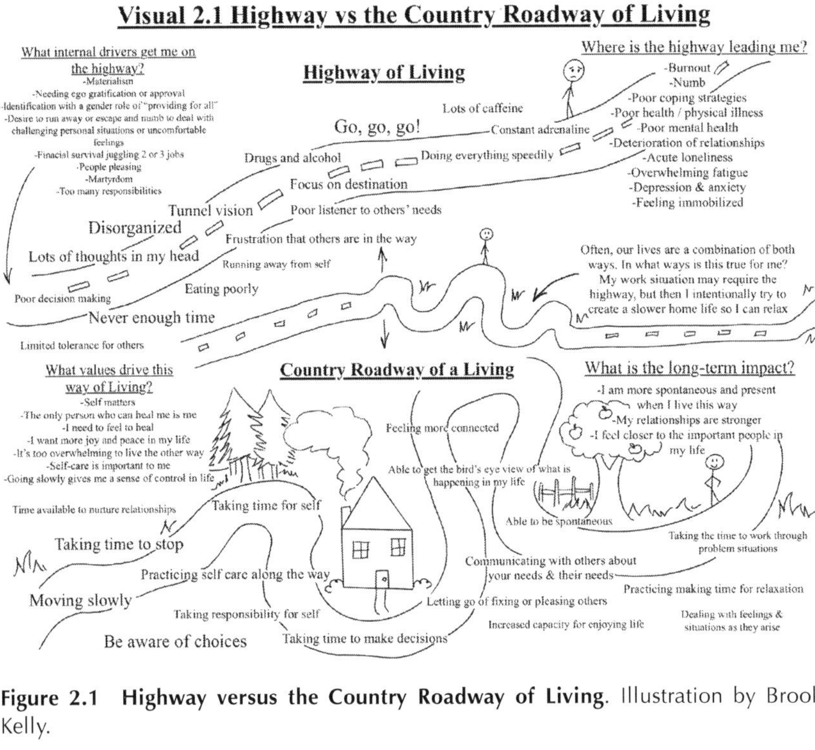

Figure 2.1 **Highway versus the Country Roadway of Living**. Illustration by Brooke Kelly.

many clients who can afford to live a more slow-paced lifestyle are often caught up in the unconscious demands of a society that values speed and speed filled living. Many clients have reported that this visual helped them to step outside of the unconscious dictates of excess materialism, people pleasing, seeking external approval through excess work, martyrdom, and other drivers. The tool starts by drawing a highway and naming it as the "highway of living."

Some questions to use to fill in the image are:

1. What are some of the characteristics of your life if you are living your life as if it is a highway? Clients have responded with descriptors such as, lots of thoughts in my head, never enough time, tunnel vision, frustration that others are in the way, focus on destination, go, go, go, doing everything speedily, adrenaline, eating poorly, lots of caffeine, drugs, and alcohol, limited tolerance for others, poor listening to other's needs, consumed by busyness, disorganized, lots of sugar to keep going, not stopping, running away from self and impulsive decision making to name a few.

2. Asking the group members: What life on the highway is leading to: some examples may be burnout, numb, poor coping strategies, poor health or physical illness, poor mental health, deterioration of relationships. acute loneliness, and symptoms of exhaustion such as overwhelming fatigue, depression, anxiety, panic attacks, and feeling immobilized.

3. Ask the group members next: What are some of the internal drivers that get you living on the highway? Answers maybe materialism, seeking approval, people pleasing, high self-expectations, cultural expectations of success, martyrdom and need to be needed, external and family expec-tations, need to survive financially and economic circumstances, needing ego gratification or approval, identification with gender role of providing for all and desire to run away or escape and numb to deal with challeng-ing personal situations, or uncomfortable feelings.

4. Now the next piece to focus on is draw a windy road and name it the Country roadway of living. Now brainstorm with the group: When you are living your life as if it is a country road what are some of the characteristics of that way of living? Answers may include time to stop, moving slowly, taking time for self, practicing self-care along the way, taking time to make decisions, be aware of choices, communicating with others re your needs and their needs, letting go of fixing or pleasing others, taking responsibility for self, time available to nurture relationships, able to get a bird's-eye view of what is happening in my life, making time for relaxation, dealing with feelings and situations as they arise, feeling more connected, more able to be spontaneous, increased capacity for enjoying life, and take the time to work through problem situations.

5. The next question to ask group members is: What values drive this way of living and what is the long-term impact? Group members may mention, self-matters, the only person that can heal me is me, I need to feel to heal, I want more joy and peace in my life, it's too overwhelming to live the other way, self-care is important to me, going slowly gives me a sense of control in life, I am more spontaneous and present when I live this way, my relationships are stronger, and I feel closer to the important people in my life.

Another piece to add to the drawing and to discuss with the group is that most of our lives are a bit of both and not either/or. Adding to the drawing a bit of both in the middle of the drawing is helpful for instance, a straight line and a curvy line, and repeat it across the page. Then making the point that perhaps your work situation requires some time on the highway, and one intentionally uses home life to off-set the stress build up with intentional relaxation, and a slower way of living outside of work. Asking the group members what else could reflect this combined way of living.

At the end of the group, I read a quote from the Dalai Lama, the quote is in response to him being asked what surprised him most about humanity.

The Body talks

This image is a powerful addition to the Deepening self-connection group as it is inviting members to connect somatically, and helping them tune into "sensations as a way of knowing" and observe what is happening in terms of sensation/tension and surfacing emotion. Clients, a week later, have reported an increased awareness of their body overall and more awareness of their feelings after integrating this groups' visual. Start by drawing a body on the board.

Some questions to use to fill in the image are:

1. Where do you feel tension or sensation in your body? As group members give ideas fill in that area with a red pen, indicating an area of tension or sensation in their body. Typical areas include neck and shoulders, tightness in the chest, back pain, constriction in the stomach, stiff jawline; but clients have also mentioned eyes, head pain, throat, knees, and fingers essentially anywhere the body chooses to store embodied emotion.
2. Once you have filled in all the areas that group members feel stress and tension, now ask the group members what feelings they tend to feel on a regular basis? Name the area of the body they feel the feeling. Fill in the feelings with red dots and use an arrow onto the open page to name the feeling. The feelings could include hurt in the chest, anxiety, fear, nervousness in the stomach, out of control feelings in the jaw, and

Visual 2.2 The Body Talks

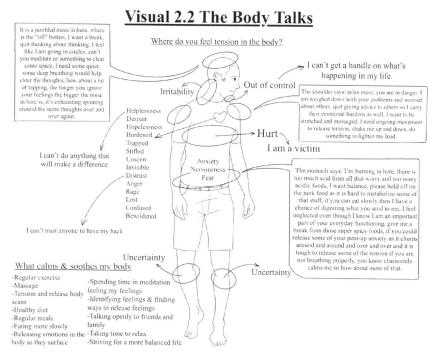

Where do you feel tension in the body?

It is a jumbled mess in here, where is the "off" button, I want a break, quit thinking about thinking, I feel like I am going in circles, can't you meditate or something to clear some space, I need some quiet, some deep breathing would help clear the thoughts, how about a bit of tapping, the longer you ignore your feelings the bigger the noise in here, it's exhausting spinning around the same thoughts over and over again.

I can't get a handle on what's happening in my life

Out of control

Irritability

The shoulder says: relax more, you are in danger, I am weighed down with your problems and worried about others, quit giving advice to others so I carry their emotional burdens as well, I want to be stretched and massaged, I need ongoing movement to release tension, shake me up and down, do something to lighten my load.

Helplessness
Despair
Hopelessness
Burdened
Trapped
Stifled
Unseen
Invisible
Distrust
Anger
Rage
Lost
Confused
Bewildered

Hurt

I am a victim

Anxiety
Nervousness
Fear

I can't do anything that will make a difference

The stomach says: I'm burning in here, there is too much acid from all that worry and too many acidic foods, I want balance, please hold off on that stuff, if you can eat slowly then I have a chance of digesting what you send to me, I feel neglected even though I know I am an important part of your everyday functioning, give me a break from those super spicy foods, if you could release some of your pent-up anxiety as it churns around and around and over and over and it is tough to release some of the tension if you are not breathing properly, you know chamomile calms me so how about more of that.

I can't trust anyone to have my back

Uncertainty

Uncertainty

What calms & soothes my body

-Regular exercise
-Massage
-Tension and release body scans
-Healthy diet
-Regular meals
-Eating more slowly
-Releasing emotions in the body as they surface

-Spending time in meditation feeling my feelings
-Identifying feelings & finding ways to release feelings
-Talking openly to friends and family
-Taking time to relax
-Striving for a more balanced life

Figure 2.2   The Body Talks. Illustration by Brooke Kelly.

uncertainty in the knees. Group members may not be able to name where they feel the feeling in their body but are aware of other feelings, for instance, helplessness, hopelessness, despair, burdened, trapped, stifled, unseen, invisible, distrust, anger, irritability, rage, lost, confused, and bewildered. Including all the feelings in the drawing is key so clients can get a sense of embodied emotion trapped in the body.

3. Next choose some of the feelings and brainstorm with the group what thoughts may be triggered by the feelings they named. For instance, with out of control in the jaw the thought may be, "I can't get a handle on what's happening in my life." For the feeling of helplessness, "I can't do anything that will make a difference" and for distrust, "I can't trust anyone to have my back." Once you have brainstormed a range of thoughts that link to the feelings it is helpful to reflect on core beliefs. If someone had these embodied feelings and some of the named repeated thoughts, What core beliefs may have formed that influences the way they see the world around them?

4. The next step is to ask the group to focus on different areas in the body. With a specific area ask the group to imagine: What that part of your

body may be communicating by the tension/sensation and/or constriction they feel? For example, if the group members mentioned their shoulders, now put a bubble from the shoulders to the open page and fill in any imagined messages from the shoulders, the messages could be, relax more, you are in danger, I am weighed down with your problems and worries about others, quit giving advice to others so I carry their emotional burdens as well, I want to be stretched, massaged, I need ongoing movement to release tension, shake me up and down, do something to help me lighten my load. Another bubble could be attached to the head and an imagined conversation from the head could be, it is a jumbled mess in here, where is the "off" button, I want a break, quit thinking about thinking I feel like I am going in circles, can't you meditate or something to clear some space, I need space, I need some quiet, some deep breathing would help me clear the thoughts, how about a bit of tapping, the longer you ignore your feelings the bigger the noise in here and its exhausting spinning around the same thoughts over and over again. Another example could be imagining what the stomach may be saying as it is gurgling in distress, I'm burning in here, there is too much acid from all that worry and too many acidic foods, I want balance, please hold off on the junk food it is hard to metabolize some of that stuff, if you can eat slowly then I have a chance of digesting what you send to me, I feel neglected even though I know I am an important part of your everyday functioning. Give me a break from some of those super spicy foods, I can't settle for days after your binges on chili peppers. Also, if you could release some of your pent-up anxiety because it churns around repeatedly and it is tough to release some of the tension if you are not breathing. You know chamomile calms me so how about more of that.

5. For a final brainstorm the group could reflect on a list of action steps that help calm and soothe the body. The heading of "what calms and soothes my body" on the open page and then members add to the list. It could include, regular exercise, massage, tension and release body scans, healthy diet, regular meals, eating more slowly and with more presence, releasing emotion in the body as it surfaces, spending time in meditation feeling my feelings, identifying them, and finding ways to release feelings. Talking openly to friends and family, taking time to relax, striving for a more balanced life, stretching that helps release pockets of tension.

Present or Past/Future

This image is particularly helpful to assist group members to become more aware if they are focusing on the past or anticipating the future, and the

Visual 2.3 Past/Future vs Present

"Be where you are otherwise you will miss most of your life."

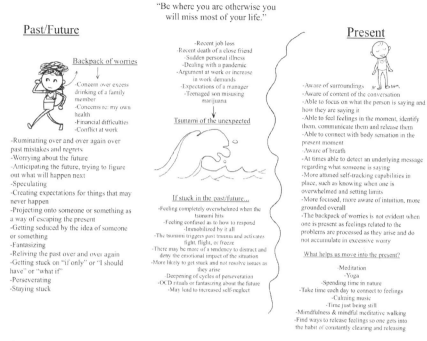

Past/Future

Backpack of worries

-Concern over excess drinking of a family member
-Concerns re: my own health
-Financial difficulties
-Conflict at work

-Ruminating over and over again over past mistakes and regrets
-Worrying about the future
-Anticipating the future, trying to figure out what will happen next
-Speculating
-Creating expectations for things that may never happen
-Projecting onto someone or something as a way of escaping the present
-Getting seduced by the idea of someone or something
-Fantasizing
-Reliving the past over and over again
-Getting stuck on "if only" or "I should have" or "what if"
-Perseverating
-Staying stuck

-Recent job loss
-Recent death of a close friend
-Sudden personal illness
-Dealing with a pandemic
-Argument at work or increase in work demands
-Expectations of a manager
-Teenaged son misusing marijuana

Tsunami of the unexpected

If stuck in the past/future...

-Feeling completely overwhelmed when the tsunami hits
-Feeling confused as to how to respond
-Immobilized by it all
-The tsunami triggers past trauma and activates fight, flight, or freeze
-There may be more of a tendency to distract and deny the emotional impact of the situation
-More likely to get stuck and not resolve issues as they arise
-Deepening of cycles of perseveration
-OCD rituals or fantasizing about the future
-May lead to increased self-neglect

Present

-Aware of surroundings
-Aware of content of the conversation
-Able to focus on what the person is saying and how they are saying it
-Able to feel feelings in the moment, identify them, communicate them and release them
-Able to connect with body sensation in the present moment
-Aware of breath
-At times able to detect an underlying message regarding what someone is saying
-More attuned self-tracking capabilities in place, such as knowing when one is overwhelmed and setting limits
-More focused, more aware of intuition, more grounded overall
-The backpack of worries is not evident when one is present as feelings related to the problems are processed as they arise and do not accumulate in excessive worry

What helps us move into the present?

-Meditation
-Yoga
-Spending time in nature
-Take time each day to connect to feelings
-Calming music
-Time just being still
-Mindfulness & mindful meditative walking
-Find ways to release feelings so one gets into the habit of constantly clearing and releasing

Figure 2.3   Past/Future versus Present. Illustration by Brooke Kelly.

impact that it has on their capacity for peace and presence. It is another essential element of the Deepening self-connection group. On a piece of paper put two columns, one area is titled Past/Future and the other Present.

1. Start the process by focusing on the Past/Future column and ask group members: How do you know you are reliving the past or anticipating the future? Group members may say, ruminating over past mistakes and regrets, worrying about the future, anticipating the future, trying to figure out what will happen next, speculating, creating expectations for things that may never happen, projecting onto someone or something as a way of escaping the present, fantasizing, reliving the past over and over again, getting stuck on "if only" or "I should have" or "what if," perseverating and staying stuck. Now put a figure at the top of the list alongside the heading; put a heart on the figure and put some walls around the heart and dizzying circles around the head to indicate disconnection from feelings and overwhelmed by thoughts. Also add a backpack onto the figure and call it a backpack of worries. It may be helpful to list some of the

stones in the backpack representing worries, for example, concern over excessive drinking by a family member, concern re own health, financial difficulties, and conflict at work to name a few.

2. For the next question ask group members: How do you know you are present and focused on the here and now? The answers might be, aware of surroundings, aware of content of the conversation, able to focus on what the person is saying and how they are saying it, able to feel feelings in the moment, identifying feelings, communicate, and release them. Able to connect with body sensation in the present moment, aware of breath, at times able to detect an underlying message regarding what someone is saying, more attuned self-tracking capabilities in place, for instance, knowing when one is overwhelmed and setting limits. Also being more focused, more aware of intuition, and more grounded overall. The backpack of worries is not evident when one is present, feelings related to the problems are processed as they arise and so do not accumulate in excessive worry. Capacity to let go is more evident in the present moment, able to tackle the concerns as they come up, and let go of aspects of problems I can't change.

3. The next development in the drawing is to draw a large wave, named "tsunami," in the middle of the drawing, stating that so often in our lives the unexpected happens and we find ourselves dealing with a whole bunch of issues all at once. Now ask the clients what the tsunami represents in their lives. It could be, recent job loss, recent death of a close friend, sudden personal illness, dealing with a pandemic, dealing with increased work demands, challenges with teenage son who is misusing marijuana, argument with work colleague, expectation of a manager, and so on. Now ask the group members what the implications are of being primarily in the past/future on one's capacity to deal with a tsunami. Responses may be feeling completely overwhelmed and confused as to how to respond, immobilized by it all, it may trigger past trauma and activate fight, flight, disassociation or freeze, there may be more of a tendency to distract and deny the emotional impact of the situation, more likely to get stuck and not resolve issues as they arise, it may deepen the cycles of perseveration, obsessive-compulsive rituals, or fantasizing about the future. Overall, it may lead to increased self-neglect.

4. The last step to brainstorm with the group is: What are some actions they can take to increasingly move into the present and away from being stuck in the past or future? A list of actions could be, increased meditation, yoga, spend more time in nature, take time each day to connect with feelings, find ways to release feelings so one gets into the habit of constantly clearing and releasing, observe patterns of behavior that let you know you are avoiding dealing with issues, observe thoughts and

discern if possible what feelings may be driving the thoughts and release them, being aware of body sensation and tension throughout the day and sense if there is an underlying feeling. Calming music, time just being still, do as many daily actions as possible practicing mindfulness and mindful meditative walking.

A quote that I introduce with this image is "be where you are otherwise you will miss most of your life" (Kornfield, 1994).

The Power of Choice

This is the fifth image in the Deepening-self connection group series. This visual can be very helpful in highlighting choice, undermining a feeling of victimization to life's circumstances, and building awareness of behaviors that undermine progress. Begin the tool by drawing a figure side on, moving down the "road of life." The figure is looking ahead.

Some questions to use to fill in the image are:

1. Draw a heart on the person and describe what they are feeling prior to a choice point in their life. It could include, relaxed, optimism, focused,

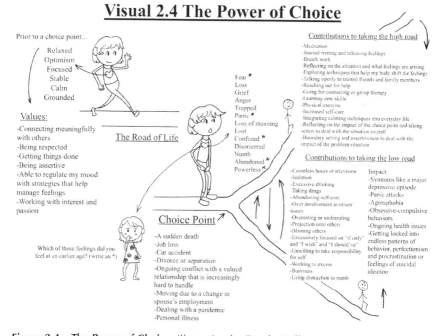

Figure 2.4   The Power of Choice. Illustration by Brooke Kelly.

stable, calm, and somewhat grounded. Another question to ask is: What are some values that guide your day-to-day life? Some responses may be, connect meaningfully with others, to be respected, to get things done, to be assertive, to be able to regulate my mood with strategies that help manage feelings, and to work with interest and passion.

2. Now indicate that the figure is further down the road of life and comes up against a "choice point." This can be a set of circumstances in our life that is forcing change at a deep level. Indicate the choice point with a crossroads. One path is moving away from the choice point to go higher and the other path moving to lower ground. A choice point could be, a sudden death, the loss of a job, a car accident, divorce or separation, ongoing conflict with a valued relationship that is increasingly hard to handle, moving due to a change in spouse's employment, dealing with a pandemic and its implications, and personal illness to name a few.

3. Draw a heart on the image and brainstorm with the group the emotional impact of the circumstances around the choice point. The feelings could be, fear, loss, grief, anger, trapped, panic, loss of meaning, lost, confused, destabilized, disoriented, numb, abandoned, stunned, powerless, and helpless. Now draw a small figure under the figure at the choice point and ask the group: Which of these feelings did you feel earlier on in your life? Link those feelings to the small figure drawing, indicating potential past trauma in the form of embodied emotion.

4. Now brainstorm with the group all the actions or inactions that contribute to moving on the low road of life. Put these actions on a road going down from the choice point forming the low road, the actions could include, countless hours of television, isolation, excessive drinking, taking drugs, abandoning self-care, over-involvement in others issues, overeating or undereating, projection onto others, blaming others, excessively focused on "if only" or "I wish" or I should've, unwilling to take responsibility for self, working to excess, busyness, using distraction intentionally to numb and cerebral communication. Taking time to reflect with the group what the impact of these behaviors could be long term. It could include symptoms such as a major depressive episode, panic attacks, agoraphobia, obsessive-compulsive behaviors, ongoing health issues, getting locked into an endless pattern of behavior, for instance perfectionism or procrastination, or feelings of suicidal ideation that are challenging to shift.

5. Now ask the group to reflect on: What actions are you taking when you move onto a higher road in life and deal with the emotional impact of the choice point? Put their answers on a road going higher from the choice point on their drawing. They may say journal writing and releasing feelings, breathwork, meditation, reflecting on the situation and what

feelings are arising, exploring techniques that help my body shift the feelings, talking openly to trusted friends and family members, reaching out for help, going for counseling or group therapy, learning new skills, physical exercise, increased self-care, integrating calming techniques into everyday life, reflecting on the impact of the choice point and taking action to deal with the situation overall, for instance boundary setting and assertiveness to deal with the impact of the problem situation.

Expansion or Contraction

This is the last in the series of visual images for the Deepening self-connection group. Heart expansion is critical to the growth process; it is indicative of "feeling feelings" at that moment in time and releasing them through a variety of methods. This visual is very similar to shrinking heart versus expanding heart in the individual section and is slightly different due to a group process. It is in the releasing of embodied emotion that unhelpful patterns of behavior are somewhat reduced, and their vice grip on our psyche lessened as another layer may have been released. In any process of change it is to be expected

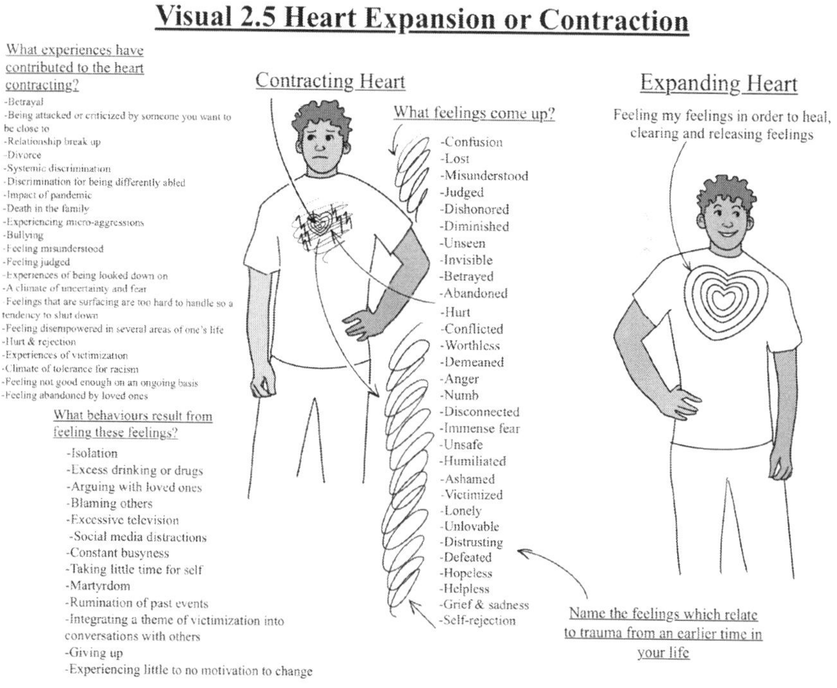

Visual 2.5 Heart Expansion or Contraction

What experiences have contributed to the heart contracting?
- Betrayal
- Being attacked or criticized by someone you want to be close to
- Relationship break up
- Divorce
- Systemic discrimination
- Discrimination for being differently abled
- Impact of pandemic
- Death in the family
- Experiencing micro-aggressions
- Bullying
- Feeling misunderstood
- Feeling judged
- Experiences of being looked down on
- A climate of uncertainty and fear
- Feelings that are surfacing are too hard to handle so a tendency to shut down
- Feeling disempowered in several areas of one's life
- Hurt & rejection
- Experiences of victimization
- Climate of tolerance for racism
- Feeling not good enough on an ongoing basis
- Feeling abandoned by loved ones

What behaviours result from feeling these feelings?
- Isolation
- Excess drinking or drugs
- Arguing with loved ones
- Blaming others
- Excessive television
- Social media distractions
- Constant busyness
- Taking little time for self
- Martyrdom
- Rumination of past events
- Integrating a theme of victimization into conversations with others
- Giving up
- Experiencing little to no motivation to change

Contracting Heart

What feelings come up?
- Confusion
- Lost
- Misunderstood
- Judged
- Dishonored
- Diminished
- Unseen
- Invisible
- Betrayed
- Abandoned
- Hurt
- Conflicted
- Worthless
- Demeaned
- Anger
- Numb
- Disconnected
- Immense fear
- Unsafe
- Humiliated
- Ashamed
- Victimized
- Lonely
- Unlovable
- Distrusting
- Defeated
- Hopeless
- Helpless
- Grief & sadness
- Self-rejection

Name the feelings which relate to trauma from an earlier time in your life

Expanding Heart

Feeling my feelings in order to heal, clearing and releasing feelings

Figure 2.5 **Expansion or Contraction**. Illustration by Brooke Kelly.

we will consciously, or unconsciously, hit a hurdle that feels too much to acknowledge or tackle. At those times we can be triggered and move into victimization and retreat into heart contraction. Through awareness of triggers and the emotional impact we can tentatively take one small step toward slight expansion. Start by drawing two figures on the page, one with an ever-expanding heart, with a heart expansion title above it, and the other with a heart that shows it is contracting layer by layer and naming this image heart contraction. Starting first with heart contraction and filling in this image.

Some questions to use to fill in the image are:

1. Ask the group members: What experiences have you had that have contributed to your heart contracting? The experiences may include betrayal, being attacked or criticized by someone you want to be close to, relationship breakup, divorce, systemic discrimination, discrimination for being differently abled, impact of the pandemic, death in the family, experiencing micro-aggressions, bullying, feeling misunderstood, feeling judged, experiences of being looked down on, a climate of uncertainty and fear, feelings surfacing are too hard to handle so a tendency to shut down, feeling disempowered in several areas of one's life, hurt and rejection, experiences of victimization, climate of tolerance for racism, feeling not good enough on an ongoing basis, and feeling abandoned by loved ones.

2. The next question to pose to the group is: How has your heart been impacted by these experiences—what feelings come up? Group members may mention, confusion, lost, misunderstood, judged, dishonored, diminished, unseen, invisible, betrayed, abandoned, hurt, conflicted, worthless, demeaned, anger, numb, disconnected, immense fear, unsafe, humiliated, ashamed, victimized, lonely, alone, unlovable, distrusting, defeated, hopeless, helpless, self-rejection, grief, and sadness.

3. Put a vortex at the heart and draw circles going downward into a spiral. Draw an arrow from the vortex to the open page and name the feelings which relate to trauma from an earlier time in your life. This builds awareness re some of the emotions are more intense than others, and can take us into a deep pit internally and contribute to unhelpful and challenging behaviors.

4. Now ask the group: What behaviors result from feeling these feelings? Behaviors could include, isolation, excess drinking, taking drugs, arguing with loved ones, blaming others, excessive television or other social media distractions, constant busyness, taking too little time for self, martyrdom, rumination of past events, integrating a theme of victimization into conversations with others, giving up, and experiencing little to no motivation to change.

For the Deepening self-connection group series, the above six images can be utilized sequentially. They can also be utilized separately for a client whose present process would be a good fit for the image. Over the years using these visuals for the six-session group I have witnessed the impact both sequentially and on their own. The key learning components of the images are all critical to a healing process and build on each other. for instance deepen self-connection, slowing down and take time to know self, connect with your body, move more into the present moment, be aware of choices and their impact, and actively expand your heart for growth. I would reiterate the themes periodically in the group and explain how they relate to the healing process. I would also include the information below in a handout as an adjunct to the group.

Healing

To heal we often need to change our lifestyle from one of perpetual busyness and distraction to slow conscious living. To initiate healing, we are actively slowing down our lives and living more consciously, connecting with your body and breath, and striving for overall balance. The body needs a state of stillness and relaxation for challenging feelings, trapped in the body, to rise to the surface for releasing. If the feelings remain stuck in the body, they create tension which contributes to feelings of stress, anxiety, feeling overwhelmed, depression, and overall tension. When we are in a healing state, we are often releasing the pain through crying, journal writing, sharing feelings related to the pain with a trusted other, moving our body for release and doing conscious breathing as some examples.

Healing also involves increasing one's awareness around patterns in relationships with people in our lives. For example, we may be over-functioning for others and trapped in a martyrdom role, or excessively depending on others and waiting for others to fix us. We could be people pleasing so we don't state our truth or minimize it. If we want to heal fully, we need to challenge patterns that feel unhealthy and stunt our growth, with assertiveness and establishing boundaries.

Healing allows us to become the person we always wanted to be. It frees us up from often intense pain and difficulty of the past and motivates us to be the best version of ourselves, shifting and changing in a more empowered direction in our lives and striving for increased peace and inner contentment.

How to start:

1. Find a quiet time every day where you can take time to reflect—start with five minutes and then build from there. If sitting is hard without

restlessness and fidgeting, take a piece of paper and write down any feelings, you feel. For instance, I feel anxious, I feel scared and restless, I feel
sad, and so forth. Use this time to also practice deep breathing. Getting
into the habit of doing daily journal writing—What are you feeling right
now? If you are concerned that someone will read your journal, tear it up
after you have written it—it is the releasing of feelings that helps long-
term healing.

2. Develop awareness around how you spend your time. Are you running
   away from yourself? When you are aware you are distracting, see if you
   can break the cycle by sitting still and being curious about what feelings
   may be driving your behavior.

3. Reflect on your relationships—Are you in a pattern where you are doing
   most of the giving or expecting others to fix you? What other patterns
   are evident? Are you playing the martyr and sacrificing your needs
   excessively, so others get what they want? Do you share your thoughts
   more than your feelings—What stops you from being more vulnerable?
   What other pressures are influencing your choices? Once you are aware
   of an unhelpful pattern, reflect on it and decide whether you want to
   change it.

4. What pain from the past is still haunting you? If you want to release
   it write a letter to someone who has hurt you in the past—tell them
   everything you wanted to say at the time. For experiences that caused
   a lot of pain we may need to write 20 or more letters to release all the
   pain. Not sending the letters means we don't need to be arguing with this
   person anymore.

5. Are you in a rut? What is missing from your life? Try a different activity
   to shake things up. Take small risks to begin with—feeling the fear and
   doing it anyway.

6. Healing needs exercise—have you been stagnant physically? What could
   you do to get more physical movement in your life? Starting each day
   by shaking to some of your favorite music is a powerful way to release
   emotion that is stuck in the body, so are stretching, breathing, and long
   walks in nature.

Following are a list of more visual images that can be used for a theme for
group therapy and adapted to reflect where the group is at in that moment.

Projection

This tool is helpful for a group where projection is an undercurrent of the
group. It is also pertinent when clients are feeling triggered by a wide range
of events in their lives and are struggling to deal with the impact. Start by

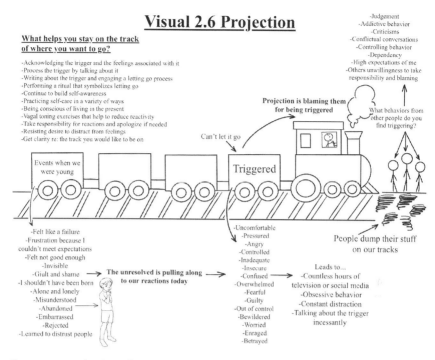

Visual 2.6 Projection

What helps you stay on the track
of where you want to go?

-Acknowledging the trigger and the feelings associated with it
-Process the trigger by talking about it
-Writing about the trigger and engaging a letting go process
-Performing a ritual that symbolizes letting go
-Continue to build self-awareness
-Practicing self-care in a variety of ways
-Being conscious of living in the present
-Vagal toning exercises that help to reduce reactivity
-Take responsibility for reactions and apologize if needed
-Resisting desire to distract from feelings
-Get clarity re: the track you would like to be on

-Judgement
-Addictive behavior
-Criticisms
-Conflictual conversations
-Controlling behavior
-Dependency
-High expectations of me
-Others unwillingness to take
responsibility and blaming

What behaviors from other people do you find triggering?

Projection is blaming them
for being triggered

Can't let it go

Triggered

Events when we were young

-Felt like a failure
-Frustration because I couldn't meet expectations
-Felt not good enough
-Invisible
-Giult and shame
-I shouldn't have been born
-Alone and lonely
-Misunderstood
-Abandoned
-Embarrassed
-Rejected
-Learned to distrust people

The unresolved is pulling along
to our reactions today

-Uncomfortable
-Pressured
-Angry
-Controlled
-Inadequate
-Insecure
-Confused
-Overwhelmed
-Fearful
-Guilty
-Out of control
-Bewildered
-Worried
-Enraged
-Betrayed

People dump their stuff on our tracks

Leads to...
-Countless hours of television or social media
-Obsessive behavior
-Constant distraction
-Talking about the trigger incessantly

Figure 2.6   Projection. Illustration by Brooke Kelly.

drawing a train on a train track towing four carriages. On the last carriage put a title of "events when we were young." On the first carriage the one linked to the train (which is symbolizing the person) put the title "triggered." Draw an arrow from the first carriage to the train and put text on the page stating projection is blaming them for being triggered. On the track in front of the train draw three stick figures and put a lot of squiggly circles symbolizing stuff on our tracks. Underneath the circles put an arrow and then write "people dump their stuff on our tracks." Now put an arrow linking the three figure's heads.

Some questions to use to fill in the image are:

1. With regard to the arrow above the three stick figures ask group members the question: What behaviors from other people do you find triggering? Some answers could be others judgment, others demands, criticism's, conflictual conversations, controlling behavior, others dependency, high expectations of me, others unwilling to take responsibility and blaming, poor insight, addictive behavior, poor self-control and impulsivity, not following through with commitments and not contributing a fair share to household tasks.

2. Underneath the first carriage that is named 'triggered' ask the group: What do you feel when you are triggered?" The list could include, uncomfortable, pressured, angry, controlled, inadequate, insecure, confused, overwhelmed, fearful, guilty, out of control, bewildered, worried, enraged, and betrayed. Also, asking what signs let you know you have been triggered, can't let it go, perseverating, obsessive behavior, constant distraction, countless hours of television or social media, talking about the trigger incessantly, and unable to settle.

3. Underneath the last carriage ask clients: What happened in your younger years that may be unresolved and that could be contributing to your trigger? The answers may be, felt like a failure, frustration as couldn't meet expectations, felt not good enough, invisible, guilt and shame, I shouldn't have been born, alone and lonely, misunderstood, abandoned, embarrassed, rejected, and learned to distrust people. Put a sentence underneath this carriage "the unresolved is pulling along to our reactions today." Another question to add is "What has happened in your past where the situation is familiar and may be related to an old trigger?"

4. Now putting text under the train (which symbolizes the group members) ask the group to brainstorm: What helps them to stay on the track of where they want to go? Some responses may be acknowledging the trigger and the feelings associated with it, process it by talking about it, writing about it, engaging a letting go process, for instance performing a ritual that symbolizes letting go. Continue to build self-awareness and be aware of choices when triggered, practicing self-care in a variety of ways, being conscious of living in the present, vagal toning exercises that help to reduce reactivity, take responsibility for reactions, apologize if needed, resisting desire to distract from how you feel, and get clarity re the track you would like to be on in your life to name a few.

"What should be" and "What is"

This group image can be powerful for clients who are impacted by cultural expectations, self-expectations, and expectations from their family of origin. Some of the expectations may have formed a core belief about self and contribute to a persistent feeling of inadequacy. Start the tool with a stick figure on top of a long rectangular box. On the top of the box write "What is."

Some questions to use to fill in the image are:

1. Put a huge cloud over the figure and put a heading above the cloud of "what should be." Then ask the group members what some of the expectations and beliefs are regarding who they "should be" in the world. Some potential answers are, I should be fulfilled, I should be happy, I

Visual 2.7 "What Should be" and "What is"

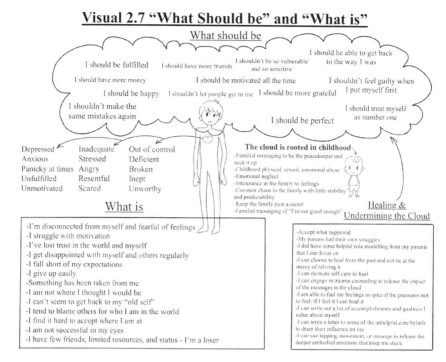

Figure 2.7 "What Should Be" and "What Is." Illustration by Brooke Kelly.

should be motivated all the time, I shouldn't make the same mistake again, I shouldn't be so vulnerable and so sensitive, I shouldn't let people get to me, I should be able to get back to the way I was, I should be perfect, I should treat myself as number one, I shouldn't feel the way I do, I shouldn't feel guilty when I put myself first, I should be more grateful, I should have more friends, money, status, more success than I have.

2. Now ask the group "what is" your present reality and put the answers in the long rectangle. Some responses may be, I'm disconnected from myself and fearful of feeling, I struggle with motivation, I've lost trust in the world and myself, I get disappointed with myself and others regularly, I fall short of my expectations, I give up easily, something has been taken from me, I am not where I thought I would be, I can't seem to get back to my "old self," I tend to blame others for who I am in the world, I find it hard to accept where I am at, I am not successful in my eyes, I have few friends, limited resources, and status, and feel like a loser sometimes.

3. Put a heart on the figure and brainstorm what feelings are generated by both lists. Put an arrow onto the open page linking the heart and write down the feelings. They may include, depressed, anxious, panicky at

times, unfulfilled, unmotivated, inadequate, stressed, angry, resentful, scared, out of control, deficient, broken, inept, unsuccessful, unworthy, helpless, hopeless, and disempowered.

4. Now draw a line linking the cloud of "what should be" to the feelings that result from the thoughts, and core beliefs about self and write alongside it "the cloud is rooted in childhood." Also draw some overarching family figures (if there is space on the page) with lines toward the arrows indicating their projections onto the child. Now draw several arrows next to the line linking the cloud to the feelings. Insert a statement with each of the arrows describing some of the family of origin pressures and experiences which contributed to high expectations of self with minimal self-compassion. Some of the statements could include familial messaging to be the peacekeeper and suck it up, experiences of childhood physical, emotional, and sexual abuse, emotional neglect, intolerance in the family to feelings, constant chaos in the family with little stability and predictability, keep the family pain a secret and familial message of unworthiness, not good enough and it's all my fault.

5. Draw a column over to the far right of the page. Title the column "Healing and undermining the cloud." Now ask the group: What helps you to heal and undermine the messages in the cloud. Some answers may be, accept what happened, my parents had their own struggles, I did have some helpful role modeling from my parents that I can focus on, I can choose to heal from the past and not be at the mercy of reliving it, I can do more self-care to heal, I can engage in trauma counseling to release the impact of the messages in the cloud, I am able to feel my feelings in spite of the pressures not to feel, if I feel it I can heal it, I can write out a list of accomplishments and qualities I value about myself, I can write a letter to some of the unhelpful core beliefs to drain their influence on me, I can write an ongoing letter to my parents (not to send) to release the hurt and pain from the past and I can use tapping, movement, and massage to release the deeper embodied emotions that keep me stuck.

The Struggle for Self-Acceptance

This drawing on self-acceptance illuminates key themes for clients in their process of healing, as the struggle for self-acceptance can be a strong barrier to growth. Start the drawing by drawing a series of intense peaks and valleys and place the client in the middle of a valley. Put a heart on the client.

Some questions to use to fill in the image are:

1. Ask the group members: When they are stuck in the valley and rejecting self what are some of the feelings they feel? Answers might be, self-loathing, self-rejection, stuck, hopeless, helpless, disconnected,

Visual 2.8 The Struggle for Self-Acceptance

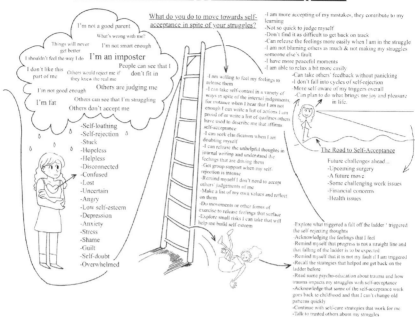

Figure 2.8   The Struggle for Self-acceptance. Illustration by Brooke Kelly.

confused, lost, uncertain, angry, low self-esteem, depression, anxiety, stress, shame, guilt, self-doubt, and overwhelmed to name a few.

2. Now place a cloud over the valley and enquire with group members: What stories in your head are intensifying the struggle to self-acceptance? The stories may include, I shouldn't feel the way I do, I'm not a good parent, things will never get better, I don't like this part of me, what's wrong with me, I'm not good enough, I don't measure up, others don't accept me, I'm fat, I'm not smart enough, people don't accept me for who I am, I'm an imposter, people can see that I don't fit in, people don't like me, others would reject me if they knew the real me, others are judging me and others see that I am struggling.

3. Now place a ladder at the foot of the person in the drawing reaching up past the highest peak. Now ask the group members: What do you do to move toward self-acceptance despite your struggle? Put an arrow from the ladder to the open page and write down the group member answers. They may include, I am willing to feel my feelings to release them, I can take self-control in a variety of ways despite the internal judgments, for instance when I hear I am not enough I can write a list of actions I am proud of, or write a list of qualities others have used to describe me

that affirm self-acceptance. I can seek clarification when I am doubt-ing myself, I can release the unhelpful thoughts in journal writing and understand the feelings that are driving them, remind myself I don't need to accept other's judgments of me, get group support when my self-rejection is intense, make a list of my own values and use those as a reflection of my accomplishments and what I value the most. Do move-ment or other forms of exercise to release feelings that surface, explore small risks that I can take that will help build self-esteem.

4. Now ask the group members: What are some strategies to get back on the ladder when you fall off that will move you toward self-acceptance? Draw a figure falling off the ladder and now include their thoughts on the open page. Group members may express as a strategy, explore what may have triggered me and triggered the self-rejecting thoughts, acknowledge the feelings that I feel, remind myself that progress is not in a straight line that falling off the ladder is to be expected, remind myself it is not my fault if I am triggered, recall the strategies that helped me get back up the ladder before, read some psycho-education about trauma and how trauma impacts my struggle with self-acceptance, acknowledge that some of the self-acceptance work goes back to childhood and that I can't change old patterning quickly, continue with self-care strategies that I know are effective for me, talk to trusted others about my struggle, and ask for feedback where it could be helpful to reduce the intense self-criticism.

5. Now draw a person out of the peaks and valleys for a while and on the bumpy road of self-acceptance, pointing out even the road of self-acceptance has bumps in it given life's challenges. Draw some more peaks and valleys in the distance but not as steep. Ask the group mem-bers: How will you know you are on the road to self-acceptance? Their answers may include, am more accepting of my mistakes, see my mis-takes as contributing to my learning, am not so quick to judge myself, don't find it as difficult to get back on track, am not as tormented by the thoughts, am able to release the feelings more easily when I am in the struggle, I am not blaming others as much and not making my struggle someone else's fault, have more peaceful moments in my life, am able to relax a bit more easily, can take others feedback and not go into a panic and a cycle of self-rejection, am more aware of self and triggers overall, can foresee some of my struggles up ahead and have some strategies to deal with them. Can plan to do what brings me joy and pleasure in life.

6. Lastly ask group members if they see foresee some challenges ahead and is there anything they can do now to prepare. Show the upcoming events with a triangle shape to the eyes moving into the future. Group members could respond with events such as upcoming surgery, a future move,

some challenging work issues, financial concerns, and health issues to name a few. The strategies may also include those already discussed.

Dealing with a Backpack of Worries and Unresolved Trauma

To start the drawing, draw a figure facing sideways at the far-left hand of the page. Now draw a large backpack on the figure and draw stones, both large and small, in the backpack; now name the stones as "present worries" and "unresolved trauma."

Some questions to use to fill in the image are:

1. Ask the group members: What is presently worrying you and what past trauma do you feel you are still carrying around? Answers could include, sexual abuse in childhood and difficult intimate relationships, past addiction in the family and experience of neglect, attacked by a stranger find it hard to feel safe, abusive husband who yells at me, being adopted and not feeling like I belong, financial concerns, distance and conflict in family, difficulty sleeping, finding it hard to get out of bed, poor motivation,

Visual 2.9 Dealing With the Backpack of Worries and Unresolved Trauma

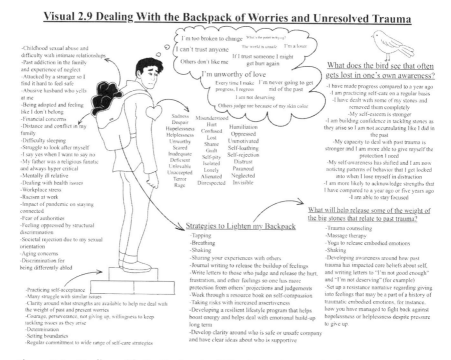

Figure 2.9 Dealing with the Backpack of Worries and Unresolved Trauma. Illustration by Brooke Kelly.

struggle to look after myself, say yes when I want to say no, father was a religious fanatic and hypercritical, mentally ill relative, dealing with health issues, finding it difficult to walk due to feet issues, impact of past drug addiction, workplace stress, isolated, impact of pandemic on staying connected, racism at work, experiencing micro-aggressions, experiencing marginalization, fear of authorities, feeling oppressed by structural discrimination, societal rejection re sexual identity, and aging concerns.

2. Now draw a heart on the figure and with an arrow onto the open page ask the group: What feelings do you feel and what feelings may be embodied due to past trauma? Their answers could include, sadness, despair, hopelessness, helplessness, unworthy, scared, inadequate, deficient, unlovable, unaccepted, terror, rage, misunderstood, hurt, confused, lost, shame, guilt, self-pity, isolated, lonely, alone, alienated, disrespected, humiliation, oppressed, unmotivated, self-loathing, self-rejection, distrust, paranoid, neglected, bewildered, invisible, and invalidation to name a few.

3. Next draw a large bubble over the head of the figure and enquire: What are some of the thoughts that you are aware of that keep your mind busy and may be related to some of the embodied emotion? Some ideas maybe, I'm too broken to change, there's something wrong with me, I can't trust anyone, others don't like me, others are out to get me, I'm unworthy of love, if I trust someone I may get hurt again, nobody gets me, the world is unsafe, I'm all alone, what's the point in trying, every time I make progress I regress, I can't do it, I'm never going to get rid of the past, others will always see me as not good enough, I'm a loser, others judge me because of my skin color, I am not deserving and no one gets me for who I am.

4. Now draw some arrows coming from the backpack and title it, Strategies to lighten my backpack. Group members are asked about their strategies, these could include, breathing, tapping, shaking, sharing your experience with others, journal writing to release the buildup of feelings, writing letters to those that judge and releasing the hurt, frustration and other feelings so one has more protection from others projections or judgments, work through a resource book on self-compassion, taking risks with increased assertiveness, develop clarity re who is safe or unsafe company, and have clear ideas about who is supportive, developing a resilient lifestyle program that helps boost energy and helps to clear some of the emotional build-up.

5. Now with a focus on the big stones in the backpack—ask the group members what strategies may be particularly helpful to release some of the big stones that relate to past trauma. Some of the strategies may be, trauma counseling, massage therapy, acupuncture, yoga to release embodied

emotion, shaking, developing awareness around how past trauma has impacted core beliefs about self and writing letters to "not good enough" or "I am not deserving" for example. Release some of the old story by acknowledging and dealing with embodied emotion related to the core beliefs. In addition, set up a resistance narrative regarding giving into feelings that may be part of a history with traumatic embodied emotions, for instance, how have you managed to fight back against hopelessness or helplessness despite pressure to give up.

6. Now put some bricks under the figure and brainstorm with the group what helps to build a firm foundation under one's feet, so a backpack doesn't destabilize us and throw us off balance. Some bricks could be practicing self-acceptance, realizing that many are struggling with similar issues, building clarity around what strengths are available to access regularly so that one can deal with the weight of the past and present worries. Some strengths may be, perseverance and courage, not giving in and a willingness to keep tackling the issues as they arise. Another strength may be determination, and clients could brainstorm how determination impacts their ability to face their issues and resolve the past. Other bricks could be ongoing assertiveness and boundary setting to those who have undermined trust in the past, and a regular commitment to a wide range of self-care strategies.

7. Lastly a bird in the top right-hand side of the drawing could indicate keeping perspective. A question for group members could be: What does the bird see that often gets lost in one's own awareness? Group members could add that I have made progress compared to a year ago, that I am practicing self-care on a regular basis, that I have dealt with some of the stones and removed them completely, my self-esteem is stronger, and I am building confidence in tackling stones as they arise, so I am not accumulating as I did in the past. My capacity to deal with past trauma is stronger and I am more able to give myself the protection I need, my self-awareness has shifted so I am now noticing patterns of behavior that I get locked into where I lose myself in distraction. I am more likely to acknowledge strengths that I have compared to a year ago, or five years ago, and I am able to stay more focused on what I want to give my attention to compared to before.

Relationship Dynamics and Their Impact

This image can assist group members develop insight and increase self-awareness around co-dependency, interdependency, and independent relationship styles, and how these relationship patterns impact their capacity to deal with past trauma and manage everyday life's challenges. Start in the

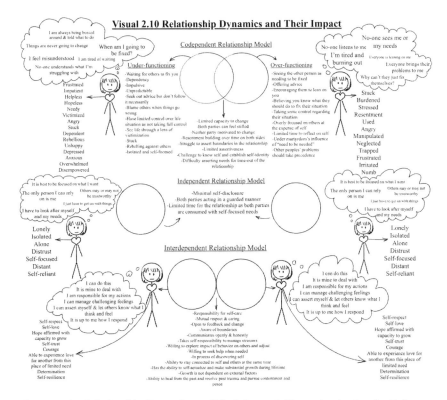

Figure 2.10   Relationship Dynamics and Their Impact. Illustration by Brooke Kelly.

middle of the page and draw two circles overlapping by about a third, put a title of Codependent relationship model. Put an arrow from the left circle and the right circle onto the open page. Below the arrow on the left write "over-functioning" and below the arrow on the right write "under-functioning." Now draw a stick figure on the side of each circle with a heart on the figure.

Some questions to use to fill in the image are:

1. Ask the group members: When you are over-functioning in relationships how would you describe your behavior regarding the other person? Answers might be, seeing the other person as needing to be fixed, offering advice, encouraging them to lean on you, believing you know what they should do to fix their situation, taking some control regarding their situation, overly focused on others at the expense of self, limited time to reflect on self, educating others that you don't have needs consciously or unconsciously, under martyrdom's influence of "need to be needed," and believe other people's problems should take precedence. Now ask the

group: If you are an over-functioner what are some of the feelings you feel? The group answers could be, stuck, burdened, stressed, resentment, used, angry, manipulated, neglected, trapped, frustrated, irritated, and numb. Now add a cloud to the head of the figure and brainstorm some thoughts the over-functioner may think regularly. They may be, no one listens to me, everyone is leaning on me, no one sees me or my needs, everyone brings their problems to me, I'm tired and burning out, and why can't they just fix themselves.

2. Now brainstorm with the group: When you are under-functioning in relationship what are some of your behaviors and feelings? The descriptors for an under-functioner could include, waiting for others to fix you, dependency, impulsive, unpredictable, seek out advice but don't follow it necessarily, blame others when things go wrong, have limited control over one's life situation as not taking full control, see life through a lens of victimization, stuck, rebelling against others, isolated, and self-focused. The feelings could include, frustrated, impatient, helpless, hopeless, needy, victimized, angry, stuck, dependent, rebellious, unhappy, depressed, anxious, overwhelmed, and dis-empowered. Some thoughts might be, when am I going to be fixed, no one understands what I am struggling with, I am tired of waiting, I am always being bossed around and told what to do, no one is listening to me, I feel misunderstood, and things are never going to change.

3. Now put an arrow from the overlap in the two circles and describe the impact of the co-dependent relationship dynamic. Group members may mention, limited capacity to change, both parties can feel stifled, neither party motivated to change, resentment building over time on both sides, struggle to assert boundaries in the relationship, limited assertiveness, challenge to know self and establish self-identity, difficulty asserting needs for a brief time-out of the relationship. I mention to clients that this can lead to an overall feeling of stable misery. Many clients relate to that term, and make the connection between boundaries being violated in childhood and a possible familiarity with stable misery. Attaching to stable misery can be a reminder of an earlier time in life when choices were not available. A time when traumatic experiences may have been experienced and there were enormous challenges in dealing with it as a child, and consequently immobilization may have been an automatic response. A conversation with clients around seeking out "the familiar" in life and that often fear of change, and the unknown path, can contribute to being locked into a co-dependent dynamic for decades. Also, worth mentioning is that the dynamic has an impact on communication in the relationship. For example, communication in the relationship can often be scripted around fixed roles, for instance it may be rare for the

over-functioner to express a wide range of feelings and seek support from a dependent partner.

4. Now put two circles below the co-dependent dynamic drawing both very wide apart. Title this drawing the Independent relationship model. Put a figure on either side of the circles and ask group members about feelings both figures may be feeling and what thoughts they may be having co-existing in this relationship dynamic. Draw a heart on both figures and repeat the feelings and thoughts for both sides. Feelings may be lonely, alone, isolated, distrust, self-focused, distant, and self-reliant. Thoughts may be, the only person I can rely on is me, I must look after myself and my needs, I just must get on with things, others may or may not be trustworthy, others can pull me down if I let them get too close, and it's best to be focused on what I want. Again, with an arrow add the impact on communication patterns in the relationship. Most often the communication pattern is minimal self-disclosure, both parties could be acting in a guarded manner and demonstrate limited time for the relationship, both parties consumed with self-focused needs.

5. The last relationship dynamic to explore with the group is the Interdependent relationship dynamic. Draw two circles both connecting at the center of the circle with no overlap; the two circles are side by side. Now add two figures on either side of the drawing, and add a heart, put an arrow from the heart onto the open page for each figure. Now put an arrow going down from the area where the circles meet side by side. Ask the group to brainstorm characteristics of this relationship model. Some descriptors may be, responsibility for self, responsibility for self-care, mutual respect, mutual caring, open to feedback and change, aware of boundaries, willing to assert self to defend and articulate boundaries, communicates openly, takes self-responsibility to manage stressors, willing to explore impact of behavior on others and adjust, is willing to seek help when needed, open and honest communication, in process of discovering self, capacity to attune to others, ability to stay connected to self and to others at the same time (unless a trigger from the past leads to nervous system dysregulation), has the ability to self-actualize and make substantial growth during lifetime, growth is not dependent on external factors, ability to heal from past and able to process past traumatic experiences that haven't been metabolized and integrated. Next enquiring with the group about feelings and thoughts that may be generated from this relationship model. Link feelings to the heart of each figure to the open page and put a bubble around the head of the figure indicating thoughts. Group members may add, feeling of self-respect, feelings of self-love, hope affirmed with capacity to grow, self-trust, able to experience love for another from this place of limited need, courage,

determination, and self-resilience. Thoughts may be, I can do this, it is mine to deal with, I am responsible for my actions, I can manage challenging feelings, I can assert myself and let others know what I feel and think, and it is up to me how I respond.

Feeling's Scale—Awareness of Feelings and Releasing Feelings

Working through past trauma can trigger a wide range of sensations and embodied emotion and can trigger other symptoms of nervous system dysregulation. The client may experience reliving the event as if it is occurring right now, given the role of the amygdala-centric circuits. Given past triggers, and memories of dysregulation, clients often have developed a fear of the intensity of the feelings they feel at times. Also, with intense feeling states the client may move outside their window of tolerance and shut down in hypoarousal, therefore a prevalent feeling can be numb or feeling disconnected. This visual can help normalize emotional responses and the intensity of emotion, challenge cultural pressures to not feel feelings and to

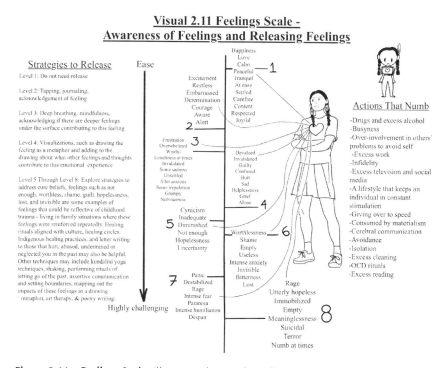

**Visual 2.11 Feelings Scale -
Awareness of Feelings and Releasing Feelings**

Figure 2.11   Feelings Scale. Illustration by Brooke Kelly.

mask inner experiences, and give some ideas regarding strategies for dealing with different feelings.

Start the drawing with a vertical line down the middle of the board or paper. Now mark short horizontal lines at regular intervals putting 1 – 8 on the line. Draw a figure on the right-hand side of the page with a heart and link the emotions on each level to the heart. Also draw on the other side of the scale a long vertical line with an arrow that indicates ease regarding feeling feelings at the top of the line, and at the end of the line indicate feelings that are highly challenging to feel and may lead to numbing strategies. Have space at the left side of the page to list "strategies to release" and on the far-right "actions that numb" and lead to disconnection from self. Put a figure above the title "actions that numb" and put a heart on the figure and walls around the heart to indicate numbing.

Some questions to use to fill in the image are:

1. Ask the group members what feelings they feel at every level. Encourage the group members to give a rating of depth according to their own experience, there may be significant differences in the group whereby one group member is able to tolerate anger more easily for instance than another. The point of the scale is to assist group members to start to rate their own feelings for intensity and to build awareness around which feelings are the most challenging for them. The scale is primarily focused on challenging feelings because of their capacity to trigger dysregulation. It can be helpful for clients to note which feelings are a trigger of past traumatic memories. Level 1 are feelings that are comfortable to feel. What feelings do you feel when you are at Level 1 on the scale? Clients may mention, love, happy, calm, peaceful, tranquil, at ease, settled, carefree, content, respected, and joyful. Level 2 feelings may be, excited, restless, embarrassed, determination, courage, aware, and alert. For Level 3 feelings the group could include, overwhelmed, wistful, loneliness at times, invalidated, some sadness, unsettled, some trepidation, a bit anxious, anticipation, nervousness, grumpy, and frustration. Level 4 feelings could be described as, devalued, invalidated, guilty, confused, hurt, sad, helplessness, grief, and alone. Level 5 feelings may be inadequate, diminished, not enough, hopelessness, cynicism, and uncertainty. Level 6 feelings could be, useless, worthless, shame, empty, intense anxiety, invisible, bitterness, and lost. Level 7 feelings may include panic, destabilized, rage, intense fear, paranoia, intense humiliation, and despair. The last feelings on the scale Level 8 could include, utterly hopeless, immobilized, empty, meaninglessness, suicidal, terror, rage, and numb at times. None of the feelings on the scale are fixed; some feelings may be scaled at a lower level of intensity; for instance Level 1 to Level 3

feelings, however if any group member has a long history with a particular embodied emotion, it will likely be felt at a significantly heightened intensity and may warrant a Level 7 experience given the history. So, the feeling scale is subjective, which is why I have intentionally used phrases such as "could be" or "may be" to build in flexibility for unique individual experiences.

2. At the top of the far-left corner of the page put a title "Strategies to Release feelings." The list will vary according to the group members; however, it is helpful to have a list on the side for clients to refer to in times of distress. Some group members may for instance find tapping helpful for a wide range of distress, so strategies may vary from client to client. Alongside the Level 1 feelings add in the far-left column, these feelings do not need release. Alongside the Level 2 feelings strategies could include, tapping, journal writing, and acknowledgment of feeling. Level 3 strategies may be, deep breathing, mindfulness, and acknowledging if there are deeper feelings under the surface that are contributing to the overall feeling state. At Level 4 clients may want to consider visualizations for a particular feeling or for instance, drawing out their experience in a metaphor. Level 4 may also include movement, self-massage techniques, and talking about your feelings with a trusted other or techniques already mentioned in other levels. For Level 5 to Level 8 feelings, it may be helpful to explore strategies that address core beliefs, feelings such as not enough, worthless, shame, guilt, hopeless, invisible, and lost that could be reflective of childhood trauma and living in family situations where these feelings were reinforced repeatedly. Other strategies for the more intense, protracted feelings could be letter writing to those that impacted you in the past. These are therapeutic letters and most often are not intended to be sent unless the perpetrator is able to make amends and hear fully the impact of their behavior. Clients may need to write 10, or 20 letters, to the same person peeling back each layer of embodied emotion with each letter. I have seen the impact of letter writing in a Men's anger management group; many men had childhood abuse histories with their fathers and they used letter writing to release the rage and intensity of embodied emotion they felt to learn to manage their anger in a respectful way. Other techniques include culturally aligned healing such as healing rituals aligned with culture, healing circles, Indigenous healing practices, Kundalini yoga techniques, shaking, performing rituals of letting go of the past, assertive communication and setting boundaries, particularly with those that hurt us in the past, a full mapping out of the impact of these feelings in a drawing/metaphor (Experiential Unity model). Some clients find other forms of art therapy or creative expression helpful for releasing past pain. I have witnessed clients write poetry,

prose and sing songs, and use other forms of creativity to work through some of the pain in powerful ways.

3. In the far-left-hand column also write down all the numbing strategies that are often habitual and challenging to resist. The numbing strategies could relate to all the feelings in Level 2 to Level 8, it will be dependent on the clients' historical experiences and their capacity to regulate their nervous system and stay within their window of tolerance. The actions that numb may include, drugs and excess alcohol, busyness, over-involvement in others' problems to avoid self, excess work, infidelity, excess television and social media, a lifestyle that keeps an individual in constant stimulation, giving over to speed, consumed by materialism, cerebral communication, avoidance, and isolation as some examples. Group members may also offer some unique contributions to this list. I have heard from clients that excess cleaning and obsessive-compulsive rituals are a way of numbing, and even excess reading to escape one's own life instead of facing problems and feelings.

Living under the Mushroom

As noted earlier clients with a trauma history often experience immobilization, disassociation, or other symptoms of hypoarousal and isolate to feel safe. "Living under the mushroom" can be a way of being in the world, where life is contracting according to the intensity of nervous system dysregulation. The sense of safety under the mushroom can be both reassuring and undermining; it takes the client further away from the support they might need and an opportunity to shift out of the vice grip of dysregulation given the intense feelings.

To start the visual image, begin by drawing a large mushroom in the center of the page and place a figure under the mushroom. Put a heart on the figure and an arrow from the heart onto the open page.

Some questions to use to fill in the image are:

1. Ask the group members what entices us to live life under the mushroom, what are some of the thoughts we have about our life that encourage refuge under the mushroom? Some answers might be, people don't allow me to be who I am, I can take time out to recover, it is the only time I feel safe, no one can bug me there, I am protected from those that keep taking from me or making demands that I can't fulfill, I don't want to be exposed and vulnerable, there's too much going on, there's competition all around me and I can't keep up, others see my imperfections and I feel I have to pretend that I'm coping, I feel weak right now and need a place to hide and I can do my own thing.

2. Now move to the arrow linked to the heart and explore with the group all the feelings generated by life under the mushroom. Feelings could

Visual 2.12 Living Under the Mushroom

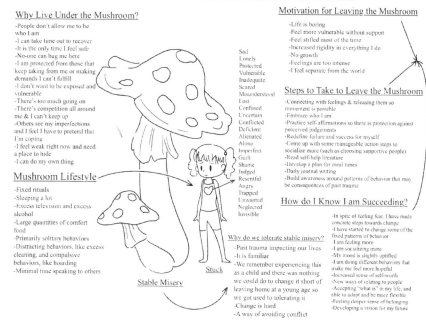

Why Live Under the Mushroom?

-People don't allow me to be who I am
-I can take time out to recover
-It is the only time I feel safe
-No-one can bug me here
-I am protected from those that keep taking from me or making demands I can't fulfill
-I don't want to be exposed and vulnerable
-There's too much going on
-There's competition all around me & I can't keep up
-Others see my imperfections and I feel I have to pretend that I'm coping
-I feel weak right now and need a place to hide
-I can do my own thing

Mushroom Lifestyle

-Fixed rituals
-Sleeping a lot
-Excess television and excess alcohol
-Large quantities of comfort food
-Primarily solitary behaviors
-Distracting behaviors, like excess cleaning, and compulsive behaviors, like hoarding
-Minimal time speaking to others

Stable Misery

Sad
Lonely
Protected
Vulnerable
Inadequate
Scared
Misunderstood
Lost
Confused
Uncertain
Conflicted
Deficient
Alienated
Alone
Imperfect
Guilt
Shame
Judged
Resentful
Angry
Trapped
Unwanted
Neglected
Invisible

Stuck

Why do we tolerate stable misery?

-Past trauma impacting our lives
-It is familiar
-We remember experiencing this as a child and there was nothing we could do to change it short of leaving home at a young age so we got used to tolerating it
-Change is hard
-A way of avoiding conflict

Motivation for Leaving the Mushroom

-Life is boring
-Feel more vulnerable without support
-Feel stifled most of the time
-Increased rigidity in everything I do
-No growth
-Feelings are too intense
-I feel separate from the world

Steps to Take to Leave the Mushroom

-Connecting with feelings & releasing them so movement is possible
-Embrace who I am
-Practice self-affirmations so there is protection against perceived judgements
-Redefine failure and success for myself
-Come up with some manageable action steps to socialize more (such as choosing supportive people)
-Read self-help literature
-Develop a plan for meal times
-Daily journal writing
-Build awareness around patterns of behavior that may be consequences of past trauma

How do I Know I am Succeeding?

-In spite of feeling fear, I have made concrete steps towards change
-I have started to change some of the fixed patterns of behavior
-I am feeling more
-I am socializing more
-My mood is slightly uplifted
-I am doing different behaviors that make me feel more hopeful
-Increased sense of self-worth
-New ways of relating to people
-Accepting "what is" in my life, and able to adapt and be more flexible
-Feeling deeper sense of belonging
-Developing a vision for my future

Figure 2.12 Living under the Mushroom. Illustration by Brooke Kelly.

include, sad, protected, lonely, vulnerable, inadequate, scared, misunderstood, lost, confused, uncertain, conflicted, deficient, alienated, alone, imperfect, exposed, guilt, shame, judged, manipulated, resentful, angry, trapped, unlovable, unwanted, neglected, and invisible.

3. Now ask the group to describe one's lifestyle living under the mushroom. It could include, fixed rituals, sleeping a lot, excess television, addictive behavior, for instance, excess alcohol and other numbing strategies like large quantities of comfort foods, primarily solitary behaviors, minimal time speaking to others, distracting behaviors and compulsive behaviors, for instance, hoarding and excess cleaning. Put a term "stable misery" under the mushroom and explore with the group if they relate to that term and why we tolerate stable misery for as long as we do? Some answers might be, it is reflective of the impact of past trauma on our lives, it is familiar, we remember a time in our lives when we experienced stable misery and there was nothing we could do as a child to change it short of leaving home at a young age, so we got used to tolerating it as a stable state hence it is familiar, change is hard, it is also a way of avoiding conflict and taking risks in life, and ritual is comforting even if it feels restrictive and stifling.

4. For the next step in the process explore with the group motivation to get out from under the mushroom. Life is boring, feel more vulnerable without support, feel stifled most of the time, increased rigidity in everything I do, no growth and feel apart from the world around me also the intensity of the feelings living under the mushroom.

5. The next question to the group focuses on steps to take to get out from under the mushroom. Group responses may be, connecting with feelings and releasing them so movement is possible, embrace who I am, practice self-affirmations so there is protection against perceived judgments, redefine failure and success for myself, come up with some manageable action steps to socialize more (choose those people who tend to be more supportive), choose one of the habits that is consuming a lot of time and make a plan to start cutting down bit by bit, start to reduce excess food intake a little and develop a plan re meal times, read self-help literature that helps with motivation, daily journal writing, build awareness around patterns of behavior that may be a consequence of past trauma, explore ways to undermine these unhelpful patterns, explore techniques that calm and soothe your body so your body is less activated during the change process, become more aware of people pleasing at the expense of self and assert self-more.

6. The last question for the group to respond to is: How do I know that I am succeeding? The list could include, in spite of feeling fear I have made concrete steps toward change, I have started to change some of the fixed patterns of behavior, I am feeling more, I am socializing more, my mood is slightly uplifted, I am doing different behaviors that make me feel more hopeful, increased sense of self-worth, new ways of relating to people, accepting of "what is" in my life, and able to adapt and be more flexible. Feeling a deeper sense of belonging with others and developing a vision for my future.

Journey up the Mountain

This visual is pertinent given clients can relate to wanting to move ahead in life and encountering obstacles, barriers, and challenges along the way. Draw a figure moving up a mountain indicating first base and second base, also indicating a peak but then a peak and valley, and peak and valley beyond that indicating that life is often filled with ongoing challenges. Also add a backpack to the figure and draw stones in the backpack representing problems encountered in life.

Some questions to use to fill in the image are:

1. Ask the group members what problems may be carried in the figures backpack, indicate problems with small stones, put an arrow onto the

Visual 2.13 Journey up the Mountain

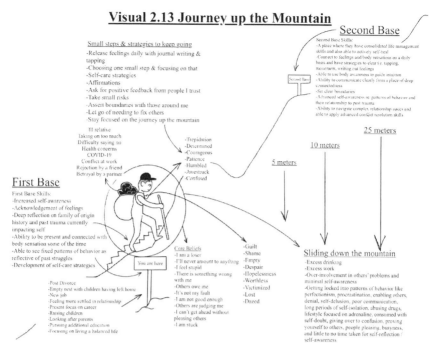

Figure 2.13 Journey up the Mountain. Illustration by Brooke Kelly.

open page, and list the problems, ill relative, difficulty saying no, taking on too much, health concerns, Covid-19, conflict at work, rejection by friend, and betrayal by partner.

2. Given where the figure is on the mountain ask the clients to brainstorm what are some of the descriptors they would use to describe where they are at in life. Put a "you are here" sign underneath their feet. Some examples might be, post-divorce, empty nest with children having left home, new job, feeling more settled in relationship, present focus on career, raising children, looking after parents, pursuing additional education, and focus on living a balanced life.

3. Ask the group what helped them to get to their first base in life, a place of progress where they can manage their life differently. Also, what skills/abilities would be reflective regarding arriving on second base on the mountain? First base skills could be, increased self-awareness, acknowledgment of feelings, deep reflections on family of origin history, and past traumatic experiences currently impacting self. Ability to be present and connected with body sensation some of the time, able to see fixed patterns of behavior as reflective of past struggles and development of self-care strategies. Now brainstorm with the group second base skills, a

place where they have consolidated life management skills and are able to actively self-heal. These could include, connected with feelings and body sensations on a daily basis and have strategies to clear for instance, movement, tapping, writing out feelings. Able to use body awareness to guide intuition, ability to communicate clearly from a place of deep connectedness, set clear boundaries, advanced self-awareness re patterns of behavior and their relationship to past trauma, and ability to navigate complex relationship issues, and apply advanced conflict resolution skills.

4. Now put a title on the open page called Sliding down the mountain. Put three arrows showing slides of different levels one may be 5 meters, another 10 meters, and the third 25 meters. Now under the title "Sliding down the mountain" ask the group participants what actions/behaviors in your life undermine your efforts and contribute to regression. Some activities could be, excess drinking, excess work, over-involvement in others problems and minimal self-awareness, getting locked into patterns of behavior like perfectionism, procrastination, enabling others, denial, self-delusion, poor communication with others, long periods of self-isolation, abusing drugs or medication, lifestyle focused on adrenaline, consumed with self-doubt, giving over to confusion, proving yourself to others, people pleasing, busyness, and little time taken for self-reflection or self-awareness.

5. Now put a circle around the climber up the mountain and link an arrow to the circle. Draw the arrow going down the mountain in the same direction as other arrows contributing to sliding down the mountain. Name the circle "core beliefs." Ask group members: What core beliefs about yourself impact you making progress up the mountain? Some answers might be, I am a loser, I'll never amount to anything, I feel stupid, there's something wrong with me, others owe me, it's not my fault, I am not good enough, others are judging me, I can't get ahead without pleasing others, I am stuck, someone needs to help me, and life is not fair.

6. Now put a heart on the figure and brainstorm feelings felt along the way, they could include, determined, courageous, scared, intimidated, overwhelmed, confused, trepidation, uncertainty, patience, humbled, small, awestruck to name a few. There may also be a range of feelings associated with sliding down the mountain including guilt, shame, despair, hopelessness, helplessness, futility, empty, gutted, trapped, stuck, inadequate, deficient, worthless, victimized, lost, disorientated, and dazed.

7. Now put some small steps on the mountain close to the climbers' feet. Name the steps, "small steps and strategies to keep going." Ask the group what strategies they use in their lives to continue to make progress despite life's challenges. The group may respond, release feelings

daily with journal writing and tapping, choosing one small step and focus on that, conscious of being present, awareness of thoughts and beliefs and how they are impacting my present abilities, self-care strategies, affirmations, acknowledge past achievements as boosting self, remind myself of my strengths that I apply to countless life situations, ask for positive feedback from people I trust, take small risks, being willing to experiment with new strategies that may or may not work, assert boundaries with those around me to maintain my power, let go of needing to please or fix others and stay focused on my journey up the mountain.

Addiction

This visual is helpful for clients who feel addictive behaviors are dominating their lives, and that they are feeling increasingly out of control with managing the addiction. Start the image by drawing a figure facing sideways with a ball and chain around each ankle. Name one ball and chain "unresolved trauma," and the other "addictions." Draw a heart on the figure.

Visual 2.14 Addiction

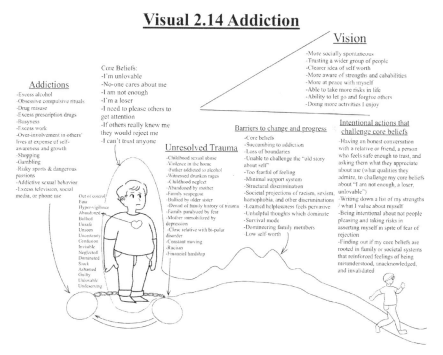

Figure 2.14   **Addiction**. Illustration by Brooke Kelly.

1. Some questions to use to fill in the image are:
2. Ask the group to name their addictions, link their answers to the ball and chain named "addictions." The answers might be, excess alcohol, obsessive-compulsive rituals, drug misuse, excess prescription drugs, busyness, excess work, over-involvement in others' lives at expense of self-awareness and growth, shopping, and other adrenaline-focused activities, such as gambling, risky sports, dangerous passions, addictive sexual behavior, excess television, and time-consuming social media or cell phone use.
3. Name the other ball and chain unresolved trauma and put a feedback loop regarding how each influences the other. Now list unresolved trauma, group members may add, childhood sexual abuse, violence at home, father addicted to alcohol, witnessed drunken rages, childhood neglect, abandoned by mother, family scapegoat, bullying by older sister, denial of family history of trauma, family paralyzed by fear, mother immobilized with depression, close relative with bipolar illness, constant moving, racism, and financial hardship.
4. Now put an arrow from the heart to the open page and list feelings associated with the trauma. Group members may state, out of control, fear, hypervigilance, abandonment, unsafe, uncertainty, confusion, invisible, neglected, unseen, bullied, pushed around, dominated, stuck, helpless, hopeless, ashamed, guilty, underserving, and unlovable.
5. Put a two-thirds circle around the figure, leave an opening in the front by the figure's feet. Now list core beliefs which are pervasive and trigger challenging thoughts as well. Some core beliefs might be, I'm unlovable, no one cares about me, I am not enough, I'm a loser, I need to please others to get attention, If others really knew me they would reject me, I can't trust anyone and no-one understands me.
6. Now put a range of squiggly lines in the opening for the path through, make the lines very high in the front and then they somewhat dissipate, but rise and fall throughout the path through. Link these barriers with an arrow to the open page and name them barriers to change and to progress. The list of barriers could include core beliefs, succumbing to addiction, loss of boundaries, unable to challenge the "old story about self," too fearful of feeling, minimal support system, structural discrimination, societal projections of racism, sexism, homophobia, and other discriminations. Learned helplessness feels pervasive, unhelpful thoughts which dominate, in survival mode in life, domineering family members, and low self-worth.
7. The next question to ask group members is: What are some specific steps on the path that challenge core beliefs with intentional action and action steps to move through barriers to progress or change? For example, if the core belief is, "I can't trust anyone," then the group member, if ready and willing, starts to take small risks in developing or

deepening friendships as a way of undermining this core belief. During this process it is critical for clients to understand any action against a core belief may well trigger turbulence as the feelings associated with the core belief, for instance, fear, distrust, paranoia, and hyper-vigilance, may be triggered. Some ideas from the group might be, have an honest conversation with a relative or friend, ask a person (whoever feels the safest) what they appreciate about you, what qualities do they admire as a way of counteracting some core beliefs around "not enough, unlovable and I'm a loser." Other ideas might be writing down a list of strengths one values in oneself. Also, being intentional around not people pleasing and taking risks in asserting oneself despite fears of rejection. Other ideas around "not being understood" could benefit from some exploratory work around where did that idea come from. At times these ideas are rooted in family systems or societal systems, understanding the participants in the system, and how the core beliefs developed and reinforced feelings of being misunderstood, unacknowledged, and invalidation. This helps in chipping away at the rigidity of the core belief and undermining its influence.

8. Ask group members to write out a list of steps they could take in the future, when ready, that would continue to chip away at rigid core beliefs and create movement and a sense of progress similar to the ones above but more specific to their situation.

9. Lastly brainstorm with group members a vision of where they would like to get to in their lives. Draw a long triangle from the figure's eyes to the open page and name it "vision." This could include more socially spontaneous, trusting a wider group of people, clearer idea of self-worth, more awareness of strengths and capabilities, more at peace with self, able to take more risks in life, ability to let go and forgive others, and doing more activities I enjoy.

Self-Doubt and Procrastination

Many clients relate to being immobilized with self-doubt and to the vice grip of procrastination. This image helps group members unpack the power of self-doubt and procrastination and explores the impact both can have on day-to-day life functioning and self-worth. Start the drawing by putting a figure in the middle of the page and put nine potential paths surrounding the figure. Each path has the word choice in it. Put a heart on the figure and circles around the top of the head to indicate "thinking about thinking" and confusion. Also draw lines from the eyes to each of the paths surrounding the figure indicating the figure is finding it hard to think straight. Also put some squiggly lines under the figure's feet indicating an ongoing earthquake, both minor and major tremors,

Visual 2.15 Self-doubt and Procrastination

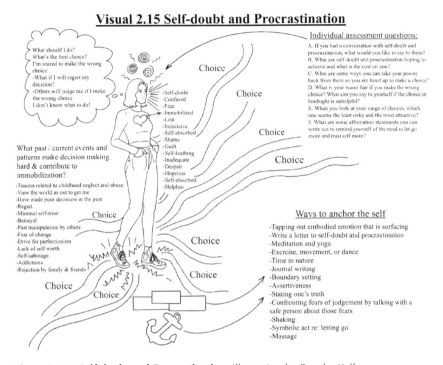

Individual assessment questions:

A. If you had a conversation with self-doubt and procrastination, what would you like to say to them?
B. What are self-doubt and procrastination hoping to achieve and what is the cost on you?
C. What are some ways you can take your power back from them so you are freed up to make a choice?
D. What is your worst fear if you make the wrong choice? What can you say to yourself if the choice in hindsight is unhelpful?
E. When you look at your range of choices, which one seems the least risky and the most attractive?
F. What are some affirmation statements you can write out to remind yourself of the need to let go more and trust self more?

What should I do?
What's the best choice?
I'm scared to make the wrong choice
-What if I will regret my decision?
-Others will judge me if I make the wrong choice
I don't know what to do!

-Self-doubt
-Confused
-Fear
-Immobilized
-Lost
-Indecisive
-Self-absorbed
-Shame
-Guilt
-Self-loathing
-Inadequate
-Despair
-Hopeless
-Self-absorbed
-Helpless

What past / current events and patterns make decision making hard & contribute to immobilization?

-Trauma related to childhood neglect and abuse
-View the world as out to get me
-Have made poor decisions in the past
-Regret
-Minimal self-trust
-Betrayal
-Past manipulation by others
-Fear of change
-Drive for perfectionism
-Lack of self worth
-Self-sabotage
-Addictions
-Rejection by family & friends

Choice

Ways to anchor the self

-Tapping out embodied emotion that is surfacing
-Write a letter to self-doubt and procrastination
-Meditation and yoga
-Exercise, movement, or dance
-Time in nature
-Journal writing
-Boundary setting
-Assertiveness
-Stating one's truth
-Confronting fears of judgement by talking with a safe person about those fears
-Shaking
-Symbolic act re: letting go
-Massage

Figure 2.15   Self-doubt and Procrastination. Illustration by Brooke Kelly.

that de-stabilizes the figure on an ongoing basis. Also put a long line with an anchor at the end of it under the earthquake and feet.

Some questions to use to fill in the image are:

1. Fill in some of the choices with the group members that they are presently grappling with in their lives.
2. Enquire with the group what events and patterns have occurred in the past and those in day-to-day life that make decision making hard and contribute to immobilization. Put the answers with the squiggly lines of an earthquake. Some answers might be, trauma related to childhood neglect and abuse, view the world as out to get me, have made poor decisions in the past, regret, minimal self-trust, betrayal, past manipulation by others, fear of change, drive for perfectionism, lack of self-worth, self-sabotage, addictions, and rejection by family and friends.
3. Ask the group members what feelings arise when self-doubt is dominant and when procrastination is making it difficult to make a decision? Some feelings may include, self-doubt, confused, fear, immobilized, lost, indecisive, self-absorbed, shame, guilt, self-loathing, inadequate, despair, hopeless, and helpless.

4. Put a cloud over the figures head and write the thoughts that are dominating. Some examples could be, what should I do, what's the best choice, what if I will regret my decision, I'm scared to make the wrong choice, others will judge me if I make the wrong choice, and I don't know what to do.

5. Now explore with the group members ways they can anchor themselves to reduce the tremors and undermine self-doubt and procrastination. Some ideas could be, tapping out embodied emotion that is surfacing, writing a letter to self-doubt and procrastination to begin to release their hold, meditation, yoga, exercise, time in nature, journal writing, boundary setting, assertiveness, stating one's truth, confronting fears of judgment by talking with a safe person about fears, movement, dance, shaking, symbolic act re letting go of challenging feelings, and massage.

6. Now if each group member can do an individual assessment of their situation by answering the following questions:
   a) If you had a conversation with self-doubt and procrastination, what would you like to say to them?
   b) What are self-doubt and procrastination hoping to achieve and what is the cost on you?
   c) What are some ways you can take your power back from them, so you are freed up to make a choice?
   d) What is your worst fear if you make the wrong choice—what can you say to yourself if the choice in hindsight is unhelpful?
   e) When you look at your range of choices which one seems the least risky and the most attractive?
   f) What are some affirmation statements you can write out to remind yourself of the need to let go and trust self more?

Stable Misery

This term encapsulates the intensity of feeling stuck and trapped that clients experience at times. The feeling can be linked to immobilization, a symptom of autonomic nervous system dysregulation, along with other symptoms of hypoarousal. I have worked with many clients where "stable misery" aptly describes the state they find themselves in; they are aware they feel stuck, trapped, paralyzed, or immobilized and also experience very little wriggle room to move and change. This image helps to unpack why we can experience this state, the complexity involved in shifting it, and some ideas re our struggle to make movement.

Start by drawing a figure stuck in a box with layers of the box around the figure. Draw a heart on the figure and put a cloud over its head to indicate consuming thoughts. Now draw a small figure near the bottom of the right

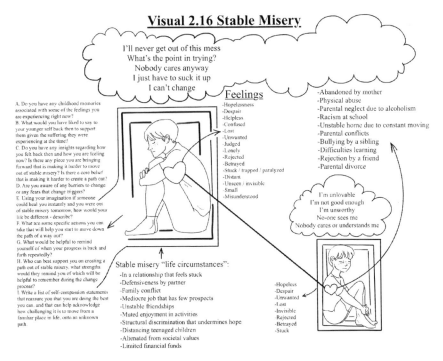

Visual 2.16 Stable Misery

I'll never get out of this mess
What's the point in trying?
Nobody cares anyway
I just have to suck it up
I can't change

Feelings
-Hopelessness
-Despair
-Helpless
-Confused
-Lost
-Unwanted
-Judged
-Lonely
-Rejected
-Betrayed
-Stuck / trapped / paralyzed
-Distant
-Unseen / invisible
-Small
-Misunderstood

-Abandoned by mother
-Physical abuse
-Parental neglect due to alcoholism
-Racism at school
-Unstable home due to constant moving
-Parental conflicts
-Bullying by a sibling
-Difficulties learning
-Rejection by a friend
-Parental divorce

I'm unlovable
I'm not good enough
I'm unworthy
No-one sees me
Nobody cares or understands me

A. Do you have any childhood memories associated with some of the feelings you are experiencing right now?
B. What would you have liked to say to your younger self back then to support them given the suffering they were experiencing at the time?
C. Do you have any insights regarding how you felt back then and how you are feeling now? Is there any piece you are bringing forward that is making it harder to move out of stable misery? Is there a core belief that is making it harder to create a path out?
D. Are you aware of any barriers to change or any fears that change triggers?
E. Using your imagination if someone could heal you instantly and you were out of stable misery tomorrow, how would your life be different - describe?
F. What are some specific actions you can take that will help you start to move down the path of a way out?
G. What would be helpful to remind yourself of when your progress is back and forth repeatedly?
H. Who can best support you on creating a path out of stable misery, what strengths would they remind you of which will be helpful to remember during the change process?
I. Write a list of self-compassion statements that reassure you that you are doing the best you can, and that can help acknowledge how challenging it is to move from a familiar place in life, onto an unknown path.

Stable misery "life circumstances":
-In a relationship that feels stuck
-Defensiveness by partner
-Family conflict
-Mediocre job that has few prospects
-Unstable friendships
-Muted enjoyment in activities
-Structural discrimination that undermines hope
-Distancing teenaged children
-Alienated from societal values
-Limited financial funds

-Hopeless
-Despair
-Unwanted
-Lost
-Invisible
-Rejected
-Betrayed
-Stuck

Figure 2.16 Stable Misery. Illustration by Brooke Kelly.

hand of the page and put the small figure in layers of a box as well. Draw a heart on the small figure and a cloud and link the heart of the adult figure to the figure of the child. Also put arrows all around the small figure indicating events and circumstances that the child experienced that added to the experience of stable misery.

Some questions to use to fill in the image are:

1. Enquire with the group members whether they relate to the term *stable misery*, if so what circumstances in their lives would explain the predicament of stable misery they find themselves in? Group members might state, in a relationship that feels stuck, defensiveness by partner, family conflict, mediocre job that has few prospects, unstable friendships, muted enjoyment in activities, structural discrimination that undermines hope, distancing teenaged children, alienated from societal values, limited financial funds, and violence in city.

2. Now ask the group members what feelings they feel in relation to stable misery? Put the term feelings out on the open page to the right and write the list of their feelings, they may mention, hopelessness,

despair, helpless, confused, lost, unwanted, judged, lonely, rejected, betrayed, stuck, trapped, paralyzed, distant, unseen, invisible, small, and misunderstood.

3. Now ask the group which of those feelings did they feel in childhood? Write out the list and link it to the heart of the younger version in a box. The group may relate to hopelessness, despair, unwanted, lost, invisible, rejected, betrayed, and stuck. Now ask the group what core beliefs emanated from these embodied emotions. They could be, I'm unlovable, I'm not good enough, I'm unworthy, no-one sees me, nobody cares or understands me.

4. Brainstorm with the group dominant thoughts and put them in the bubble above the adult version. Some thoughts mentioned maybe, what's the point in trying, nobody cares anyway, I'll never get out of this mess, I just have to suck it up and I can't change.

5. Itemize with the group the events, or circumstances, that happened to the younger version of self that contributed to the felt embodied emotion and core beliefs. Use arrows to indicate them. Group members might say parental neglect due to alcoholism, physical abuse, abandoned by mother, unstable home due to constant moving, parental conflict, racism at school, bullying by sibling, difficulties learning, rejection by friends, and parental divorce.

6. Ask group members to answer the following questions individually. The questions engage a process regarding "stable misery" and help in developing insight and a detached perspective re any actions that may help to create some change.
    a) Do you have any childhood memories associated with some of the feelings you are experiencing right now?
    b) What would you have liked to say to your younger self back then to support them given the suffering they were experiencing at the time?
    c) Do you have any insights regarding how you felt back then and how you are feeling now? Is there any piece you are bringing forward that is making it harder to move out of stable misery? Is there a core belief that is making it harder to create a path out?
    d) Are you aware of any barriers to change or any fears that change triggers?
    e) Using your imagination if someone could heal you instantly and you were out of stable misery tomorrow how would your life be different? Describe.
    f) What are some specific actions you can take that will help you start to move down the path of a way out?
    g) What would be helpful to remind yourself of when your progress is back and forth repeatedly.

h) Who can best support you on creating a path out of stable misery? What strengths would they remind you of which will be helpful to remember during the change process?

i) Write a list of self-compassion statements that reassure you that you are doing the best you can, and that help acknowledge how challenging it is to move from a familiar place in life onto an unknown path.

Chapter 4

Cultural Trends That Can Suppress and Numb Our Feelings

In the counseling process it is key to be alert to the client's lifestyle. Some of the lifestyle habits may be a consequence of traumatic experiences and ongoing nervous system dysregulation, keeping the client in activation or shutting down in a variety of ways both consciously and unconsciously. Learning about a client's lifestyle can assist in assessing client readiness to do deep work and capacity to work within their window of tolerance. Lifestyle is also a key piece to address regarding the change process. This chapter highlights some cultural trends that can create barriers to the healing process; these lifestyle habits are included in many of the drawings and are evident in the Stress pain container visual 3.1 in the disconnection column. Many clients I work with need to attend to lifestyle first, chipping away at their own pace at numbing behavior, to prime their capacity to heal and build a tolerance of feeling uncomfortable feelings. Once clients feel safe enough to connect to somatic sensation and feelings, they can explore clearing strategies for embodied emotion. This chapter explores common numbing techniques on a societal level that show up in both individual counseling and group therapy sessions.

THE BUSYNESS TREND

Henry Miller asked the question in 1945 that is overwhelmingly relevant today: "This frenzied activity which has us all, rich and poor, weak and powerful, in its grip—where is it leading us?" He continues, "There are two things in life which it seems to me all men want and very few ever get (because both of them belong to the domain of the spiritual) and they are health and freedom. The druggist, the doctor, the surgeon are all powerless to give health; money, power, security, authority do not give freedom. Education can never provide wisdom, nor churches religion, nor wealth happiness, nor security peace. What is the meaning of our activity then? To what end?" (Miller, 1945, p. 29). Busyness can be a cultural disease, and if one listens deeply to our use of language, there can be cultural pride in wearing this badge of frenzy. "Where did summer go?" is a common question. "Where did the year go? Where did the month go?"

Clients I have worked with have often articulated an underlying fear of slowing down, with an assumption that difficult feelings will arise, and so it is better to keep busy. Fear of connecting fully with self seems to drive the flurry of activity; but it leaves people feeling less and less in touch with who they are—and, in time, feeling lost. Sometimes busyness is a financial necessity and a part of financial survival; however, I have met many clients over the years with ample resources locked into busyness as a coping technique to deal with past traumatic experiences. This is profoundly disturbing because with busyness as the solution to many problems someone can live like this for decades. Moving around life like an autumn leaf that is picked up by this wind and that, forever changing direction, perhaps partners, perhaps careers or geographical location, in desperation to find that anchor from the winds of life.

Avoiding a life filled with feelings and fixating on the external world can result in an inner dialogue that is haunted by the mantra "If only." "If only I had bought that house, or put my money in shares, or married that person instead of this one, or had more children, or taken a different career—then I would be happy."

If an entire society has given over to this way of being then it's hard to buck the trend, to stop, to listen inside, to take the time to connect to oneself, to acknowledge the feelings of emptiness, the void, the meaninglessness of it all. It also becomes challenging to move at a different rhythm as there can be intense loneliness and alienation when one steps out of the whirlpool of activity and slows down. See Highway versus country road visual 2.1 to unpack some of these themes.

INFLUENCE OF TECHNOLOGY ON OUR FEELING STATE

In theory, advances in technology should be giving us more free time to connect meaningfully with others. However, it seems the opposite is occurring, and as a result, our capacity to relate to one another and to our core selves is diminishing dramatically. Television, along with social media, has people wiling away their hours engrossed in external worlds with a neglect of their internal world, and the consequent numb feelings.

Another aspect of technology is an increased exposure to violence on a screen which can trigger unconscious implicit memories and lead to nervous system dysregulation. The degree of violence that the average person is exposed to on screen is at an all-time high given video games are contributing to the impact. The American academy of Child and Adolescent Psychiatry in their research states the average American child will have watched 200,000 violent acts and 16,000 murders by the time they are 18 years old. In an article by Melinda Hawkins on how the media is desensitizing children, she quotes the American Academy of Child and Adolescent Psychiatry as stating,

> the overwhelming amount of violence seen by the typical child can desensitize him to violence by reducing his natural feelings of shock at real acts of violence, and by deteriorating his ability to empathize with victims. Violent video games also allow children to participate in what the Academy calls "virtual violence," in which they have an interactive role in creating the violent images they consume. (Hawkins, 2011, p. 2)

When an individual is numb and disconnected, they can be more susceptible to hurting and harming others, a concern I have seen repeated often in a Men's anger management group. The problem again becomes disconnection from self and all the consequent suppressed emotions that often trigger impulsive behavior.

Cell phones are also having an impact on one's ability to focus and connect to self. Many are bombarded by the constant demand of incoming messages and so it can be challenging to concentrate. Most inner work requires an intense focus and an ability to sequester the outer world to explore within. It was only 200 odd years ago that most of us spent hours wiling away our time on family farms with few distractions. The opposite is the case these days with a myriad of distractions available at one's fingertips. Sadly, this can also impact our ability to have an intimate connection with someone in our lives given our limited capacity to be focused on another. This is when technology that could improve our communication is undermining our ability to "be human" with each other. Connecting meaningfully with others is an art form like any other and is also key to the healing process. As Bonnie Badenoch states, "It is different, however, when we are with a receptive, responsive other. . . . My emerging fear and pain can be embraced by the wide window of your receptive ventral presence, and in this space, healing potentially unfolds" (Badenoch, 2018, p. 71).

In a 1993 book, *Technopoly: The Surrender of Culture to Technology*, Neil Postman imagines the impact that we are observing today. He defines a *technopoly* as a society in which technology is deified, meaning "the culture seeks its authorization in technology, finds its satisfactions in technology and takes its orders from technology" (Postman, 1993, pp. 71–72).

Speed-Filled Living

In the developed world this is overwhelmingly evident; one only needs to see the degree of patience evident in lineups in some Southern countries to note the difference. It is likely one of the reasons people go to countries with more relaxed rhythms for vacations, where they are forced to slow down, despite the internal conflict inside. Speed nowadays is seen as all good—fast food, fast cars, and speed dating. For those with a trauma background the pressure of speedy living can trigger and lead to nervous system dysregulation, given the demands of quick action and quick decision making. Speed has also taken over the way people speak. It is as if some are trying to crash all their thoughts into short time frames, because they know instinctively few people have time to really listen.

Devotion to speed fosters impatience, impatience in listening to others, hoping they get to the point quickly, impatience with messy contradictory feelings, and impatience in life in general. Malidoma Some in his book *Ritual: Power, Healing and Community* reflects on speed in the developed world. "Speed is a way to prevent ourselves from having to deal with something we do not want to face. So we run from these symptoms and their sources that are not nice to look at… I believe that the difference between the indigenous world and the industrial world has mostly to do with speed" (Some, 1993, p. 17).

Milan Kundera, a Czech writer, in his book *Slowness* states, "There is a secret bond between slowness and memory, between speed and forgetting . . . . In existential mathematics, that experience takes the form of two basic equations: the degree of slowness is directly proportional to the intensity of memory; the degree of speed is directly proportional to the intensity of forgetting" (On the virtues of slowness, 2012, p. 2).

Fixation with speed also influences the healing process profoundly. Many attend therapy sessions expecting a quick fix, somehow someone will do something to fix them, or they will have the insight of all insights, and all will be healed. Healing is often messy; implicit memories and embodied emotion are challenging to access. Accessing "sensation as a way of knowing" requires intense concentration and a willingness to explore subtleties that are often below consciousness. Some leave therapy thinking it is not for them as progress is not happening quickly enough and that they are unwilling to slow down.

Overworking

The norm of weekly work hours in the developed world is varied, going up and down according to the economy. From the time of industrialization in Britain, deemed to be the "workshop of the world," working hours were dictated by those in power. Conditions were so brutal that in 1802 a law was passed which barred certain children (those who did not live with their parents) from working more than 12 hours a day.

Regarding working through trauma, the demands of the workweek can make it extraordinarily difficult to maintain a self-connection. When one has finished a day of work it is rare that the day's tasks are finished. Parents are just gearing up for family commitments. The weekend is often barely enough time to administer life, have some social time, or recover from the exhaustion of the week. An added layer is living in cities and commuting which could be up to two hours a day. Consequently, it can be highly challenging to acknowledge sequestered feelings and unmet needs that may have accumulated for years. Necessity drives most to not contemplate any other reality, and essentially suck it up, as one needs to pay a mortgage or rent, buy food and other necessities to sustain life. This accepted norm is a significant contribution to the glaring statistics on mental health. There are staggering numbers of people on psychiatric medication, their moods a constant battleground, and their sense of core self-buried under the pile of daily demands from the world around them.

The Trend of Excess Activity

When there is trapped embodied emotion related to past trauma, individuals can be prone to behavior that is excessive, rather than balanced. The activity itself may be benign, or benign in small doses, but when done to excess it can contribute markedly to disconnection from self and a numb state. The person may enjoy running, but when they do it for long hours every day the body starts to wear out and emotionally there is a cost. Any activity of excess is at times a desire for adrenaline and the consequent escape from self. Some activities have a greater emotional cost than others; gambling is a good example, but any activity done to excess for lengthy periods can eventually lead to some sort of burnout or emotional crisis.

In my work as a group therapist, I often brainstorm with the group ways of disconnecting from feelings. The clients mention working too much or eating and sleeping too much or too little. They talk about drinking too much, taking too much medication, and watching too many movies. Some have mentioned reading, it seems benign, but clients have talked about escaping their reality through reading and that they ignore what they need to do. Others talked about excessive talking and not listening to others, blaming others repeatedly and fighting. Shopping comes up often and clients mention retail therapy gives them a short term high. Social commentator Jonathon Freedman reiterates this point: "Above the poverty level, the relationship between income and happiness is remarkably small. Yet when alternative measures of success are not available, the deep human need to be valued and respected by others is acted out through consumption. Buying things becomes a proof of self-esteem (I'm worth it chants one advertising slogan) and a means to self-acceptance" (Durning, 1991, p. 48).

Another area of excess or addictive behavior that clients talk about is "falling in love" or sexual addiction. Human relationships have become increasingly co-modified for the market through online dating sites. One is now selling oneself, talking up one's best characteristics in the hope of a date with someone special. There are also serial daters; who use dating as their drug of choice. It is the chase; the newness of the encounter, the sexual experiences with a new person, and then when messy emotions get in the way of the frivolity of it all the person is dumped. Clients recognize that the cycle in itself is the magnet, pulling themselves further and further away from who they really are and what they feel.

The Seduction of Stimulants

To survive and keep pace with a speed-filled, fast-talking world it can be helpful to have some stimulants. Coffee and alcohol are norms in today's world, and it can be hard to stick to reasonable limits. Whenever one feels exhaustion coming on, there is always caffeine. It has become the drug of choice fueling the workers to work that extra hour, that extra day, and keeping exhaustion at bay for at least a little while longer. Alcohol and drugs also contribute significantly to numbed feelings. For some it is one of the few times individuals experience relaxation and so the temptation is strong, particularly in social situations when one has lost confidence in connecting with others.

Materialism

"Early in the post-world war two age of affluence, an American retailing analyst named Victor Lebow proclaimed 'Our enormously productive economy . . . demands that we make consumption our way of life, that we convert the buying and use of goods into rituals, that we seek spiritual satisfaction, our ego satisfaction, in consumption. . . . We need things consumed, burned up, worn out, replaced, and discarded at an ever-increasing rate" (Durning, 1991, p. 45). This myth has been deeply hot-wired into the psyche of many cultures that large amounts of money will buy long-term happiness. It is not to say that one can live comfortably in poverty, but for some it is the striving for the faster car, the bigger house, the sizable boat, the expensive jewelry, that encourage those fortunate enough with financial flexibility to give away those extra hours to work, in order to satisfy the insatiable cravings of more. The more one is driven for acquisition for its own sake, the more one moves away from a sustained inner journey, and for those with trauma there can be substantial pressure to keep up and disconnect from self. Advertisers ever on the lookout to get their messages out there are creative in their bombardment. Traditionally it was television, now it is on the bank teller machine, computers, cell phones, all over public transit, even sadly in schools. Children are targeted unapologetically; they are the future to the consumer markets; and it is serious business to get across the message that one will only be truly happy if they can buy the next item of impulsive need.

Cerebral Communication

Many nowadays are so busy, so caught up in the speed of life, or responding to the latest gadgets clicks and beeps that their communication has become a waterfall of ideas. They are essentially "talking at" people rather than "talking with someone." Their minds are often full so when they meet a person willing to listen, they start to offload the latest whirlpool of thought swirling around. There is little to no feeling in their speech, rather it is often fast-paced, multi-tangential, and the rant can go on for ages. There is often a desperation to connect, but given the ideas are disconnected from feeling, it is hard to communicate at a deep level and the recipient can feel drained.

Martin Jacques in an article entitled "The death of intimacy" talks about "the very idea of what it means to be human is being eroded. The reason we no longer feel as happy as we once did is that the intimacy on which our sense of well-being rests—a product of our closest, most intimate relationships, above all in the family—is in decline" (Jacques, 2004). Along with this trend is a trend to more and more talkers and fewer listeners. A myth has developed that if we are talking, we are getting out what we need to, and we will feel better. Many a client comes to therapy with this idea. Their goal is to tell the therapist as much as possible and then somehow, they will feel better. When a client is talking at me in this way it is critical to ask the client to stop, take breaks, breathe, and resource the body as a stream of consciousness can re-traumatize and trigger the client, and consequently move them outside their window of tolerance.

CONCLUSION

Experiential Unity model, like other somatically oriented models, aligns with a right mode-oriented approach and is also committed to bottom-up processing so the clients take a strong and active role in their healing. Experiential

Unity model also integrates present-oriented somatic engagement into the therapeutic work, so the truth held in cellular memory in the body is empowered with silence, and attention to nuances of sensation, tension, feeling, and urges honor the client as the expert. This mode of working attunes practitioners to issues of power and assists them in developing a decolonial lens critical for an anti-oppressive practice. Working somatically is an important way of balancing power in the therapeutic relationship putting the client in charge, and in a position of teacher of their experience.

Another aspect emphasized by anti-oppressive practice is that clients need to be agents of their own change. Moane states,

> change is a process which individuals undergo in their own social context and through their own processes. It is fundamental that this process of change is experienced by individuals as one in which they are in control, rather than as a re-enactment of patterns of domination. . . . Developing agency is itself a central part of the liberation process. (Moane, 1999, p. 183)

Experiential Unity model aligns with the guiding principles of trauma-informed practice, including bottom-up processing, and is intent on shifting the power dynamic alluded to in an anti-oppressive practice approach in both an individual and group therapy format. It also follows other aspects of anti-oppressive practice. For example, it includes societal influences and pressures that are impacting the client in the drawings historically and in the present. Honoring these experiences assists the client in discovering all aspects of their lives, and also offers a unique critique of systemic forces the client has endured. The images are able to draw on both present somatic experience and intergenerational embodied memory, and record client interactions with systems of oppression that have impacted the client's sense of safety in the world around them. The drawings alongside the concentrated emotional experience, for example, internal conflict, also include lived experiences of marginalization, racism, systemic discrimination, abuse, confusion, hurt, alienation, grief, rejection, betrayal, and how they have influenced the way the client sees the world around them, their core beliefs, and their complex journey in working through implicit memory.

Bonnie Badenoch sums up the immense wisdom of the body and its way of guiding the healing process:

> It seems good to stop here and wonder if it is possible to begin to let go of expectations about the shape in which healing may arrive, to trust the treatment plan lying dormant and waiting within our people, to cultivate a gathering stillness so that, in the safety of the space between, healing pathways have the possibilities of revealing themselves. (Badenoch, 2018, p. 319)

To date I have felt inspired by the change I have seen in clients working through trauma with Experiential Unity model. I remain committed, and ever curious, to learn about the distinctive healing process for each person by listening deeply to their bodies' wisdom, and working with the client to map out their unique and complex experience of trauma, and history of embodiment.

References

American Group Psychotherapy Association. (2016). *Special Institute to Examine Ethics Through Theater*. https://www.agpa.org/docs/default-source/practice -resources--group-circle/2016_summer_group_circle.pdf?sfvrsn=30619fa9_2

American Psychiatric Association. (1952). *Diagnostic and Statistical Manual: Mental Disorders* (Vol. 1). American Psychiatric Association.

Andrade, J., & Feinstein, D. (2004). Energy psychology: Theory, indications, evidence. *D. Feinstein, Energy Psychology Interactive*, 199–214.

The Art of Living. (n.d.). *Bhramari Pranayama - Humming Bee Breathing*. https:// www.artofliving.org/ca-en/yoga/breathing-techniques/bhramari-pranayama

Badenoch, B. (2018). *The Heart of Trauma: Healing the Embodied Brain in the Context of Relationships. Norton Series on Interpersonal Neurobiology*. W.W. Norton & Company.

Barrett, L. F. (2016, June 3). *Are You in Despair? That's Good*. The New York Times. https://www.nytimes.com/2016/06/05/opinion/sunday/are-you-in-despair -thats-good.html

Barrett, L. F. (2017). *How Emotions Are Made: The Secret Life of the Brain*. Houghton Mifflin Harcourt.

Benor, D. J., Ledger, K., Toussaint, L., Hett, G., & Zaccaro, D. (2009). Pilot study of emotional freedom techniques, wholistic hybrid derived from eye movement desensitization and reprocessing and emotional freedom technique, and cognitive behavioral therapy for treatment of test anxiety in university students. *Explore*, 5(6), 338–340.

Boath, E., Good, R., Tsaroucha, A., Stewart, T., Pitch, S., & Boughey, A. J. (2017). Tapping your way to success: using Emotional Freedom Techniques (EFT) to reduce anxiety and improve communication skills in social work students. *Social Work Education*, 36(6), 715–730.

Bowen, Bill, Fisher, Janina, Levine, Peter A., Ogden, Pat, Porges, Stephen W., & Kolk, Bessel van der (2008a). *Body-Oriented Trauma Therapies I: Clinical Perspectives. Trauma and Fight-Flight System*. [video transcript]. Cavalcade Productions Inc. http://www.cavalcadeproductions.com/body-orientedtraumatherapy.html

Bowen, Bill, Fisher, Janina, Levine, Peter A., & Ogden, Pat (2008b). *Body-Oriented Trauma Therapies II: Clinical Perspectives. Accessing the body.* [video transcript] Cavalcade Productions Inc. http://www.cavalcadeproductions.com/body-oriente dtraumatherapy.html

Brancucci, A., Lucci, G., Mazzatenta, A., & Tommasi, L. (2009). Asymmetries of the human social brain in the visual, auditory and chemical modalities. *Philosophical Transactions of the Royal Society B: Biological Sciences, 364*(1519), 895–914.

Brattberg, G. (2008). Self-administered EFT (Emotional Freedom Techniques) in individuals with fibromyalgia: a randomized trial. *Integrative Medicine, 7*(4), 30–35.

Buczynski, R., Siegel, D., van der Kolk, B., Ogden, P., Porges, S., Lanius, R., ... & O'Hanlon, B. (2017). Transcripts of Webinar Treating Trauma Master Series. NICABM The neurobiology of trauma [Transcript]. In *The Neurobiology of Trauma - what's going on in the brain when someone experiences trauma?* https:// www.nicabm.com/program/a3-brain-trauma-fb/?del=gad1260.1.rlsa&network= g&utm_source=google&utm_medium=cpc&utm_campaign=12615923754&ad_ group_id=122845211511&utm_term=%2Btrauma&utm_content=50946125183 9&gclid=Cj0KCQiA3-yQBhD3ARIsAHuHT67l8fXUZp_lcdGAXQaMkGnoN-R4ZVwUA3ipU0vNDGb8Ni-_A9WoXE48aAuUGEALw_wcB

Canadian Policy Research Networks. (2010). Weekly hours worked and indicators of well-being in Canada, at JobQuality.ca, pp. 1–7.

Callahan, R. J. (2001). Stress, health, and the heart: A report on heart rate variability and thought field therapy including a theory of the meaning of HRV (pp.1–24). *Heart rate variability and TFT report.* https://rebprotocol.net/heartvari.pdf

Chatfield, C. (n.d.). *The Research of Candace Pert, PhD.* Healing Cancer. http://www .healingcancer.info/book/export/html/34

Cope, S. (2018). *Yoga and the Quest for the True Self.* Bantam.

Craig, G. H. (1995). *Emotional Freedom Techniques: The Manual.* Sea Ranch, CA: Author.

Dana, D. (2018). *The Polyvagal Theory in Therapy. Engaging the Rhythm of Regulation.* W.W. Norton & Company.

Diamond, J. (1978). *Behavioral Kinesiology and the Autonomic Nervous System.* New York: The Institute of Behavioral Kinesiology.

Dockett, L. (2013, April). *From Margin to Mainstream: Peter Levine's Bottom-Up Approach to Healing.* Psychotherapy Networker. https://www.psychotherapyne tworker.org/magazine/article/2346/from-margin-to-mainstream

Durning, A. (1991). How much is enough. *New Age journal* (July/August), 45–49. Adapted from the State of the World 1991, Washington, DC: Worldwatch Institute.

Field, T. A., Jones, L. K., & Russell-Chapin, L. A. (Eds.). (2017). *Neurocounseling: Brain-based Clinical Approaches.* John Wiley & Sons.

Figley, C. R., Ellis, A. E., Reuther, B. T., & Gold, S. N. (2017). The study of trauma: A historical overview. In S. N. Gold (ed.), *APA Handbook of Trauma Psychology: Foundations in Knowledge* (pp. 1–11). Washington, DC: American Psychological Association.

Fisher, J., & Ogden, P. (2009). Sensorimotor psychotherapy. In C. A. Courtois & J. D. Ford (Eds) *Treating Complex Traumatic Stress Disorders: An Evidence-based Guide*, (pp. 312–328). The Guilford Press.

Ford, J. D., & Courtois, C. A. (2014). Complex PTSD, affect dysregulation, and borderline personality disorder. *Borderline Personality Disorder and Emotion Dysregulation, 1*(1), 1–17.

Freud, S. (1962). The etiology of hysteria. In J, Strachy (Eds) *The Standard Edition of the Complete Psychological Works of Sigmund Freud*, (Vol. 3: 1893–1899): *Early Psycho-Analytic Publications* (pp. 187–221). London: Hogarth Press.

Gaesser, A. H., & Karan, O. C. (2017). A randomized controlled comparison of Emotional Freedom Technique and Cognitive-Behavioral Therapy to reduce adolescent anxiety: A pilot study. *The Journal of Alternative and Complementary Medicine, 23*(2), 102–108.

Gendlin, E. T., & Lietaer, G. (1981). On client-centered and experiential psycho-therapy: An interview with Eugene Gendlin. In *Research on Psychotherapeutic Approaches. Proceedings of the 1st European Conference on Psychotherapy Research, Trier* (Vol. 2, pp. 77–104).

Gold, S. N. (2017). *APA Handbook of Trauma Psychology: Foundations in Knowledge, Vol. 1*. American Psychological Association.

Gold, S. N. (2017). *APA Handbook of Trauma Psychology: Trauma Practice, Vol. 2* (pp. xi–599). American Psychological Association.

Goldberg, R. M., & Stephenson, J. B. (2016). Staying with the metaphor: Applying reality therapy's use of metaphors to grief counseling. *Journal of Creativity in Mental Health, 11*(1), 105–117.

Goodheart, G. J. (1975). *Applied Kinesiology. Workshop Procedure Manual*, 11th Edition. Detroit: Author.

Goodman, R. D. & Gorski, P. C. (2015). *Decolonizing "Multicultural" Counseling through Social Justice*. Springer Science + Business Media.

Grabbe, L., & Miller-Karas, E. (2018). The trauma resiliency model: a "bottom-up" intervention for trauma psychotherapy. *Journal of the American Psychiatric Nurses Association, 24*(1), 76–84.

Graham, L. (2004, January 5). *Right Brain to Right Brain Therapy*. Linda Graham, MFT. https://lindagraham-mft.net/right-brain-to-right-brain-therapy/

Graham, L. (2013). *Bouncing Back: Rewiring Your Brain for Maximum Resilience and Well-Being*. New World Library.

Greenberd, Melanie (2019). Master your feelings with new tools inspired by neuroscience. *Psychology Today Canada*. Retrieved on July, 2021 from https://www.psychologytoday.com/ca/blog/the-mindful-self-express/201906/master-your-feelings-new-tools-inspired-neuroscience

Greenberg, M. (2019, June 29). Master your feelings with new tools inspired by neuroscience. *Psychology Today*. https://www.psychologytoday.com/ca/blog/the-mindful-self-express/201906/master-your-feelings-new-tools-inspired-neuroscience

Hamilton, D. R. (2014, June 30). *5 Reasons Why You Should Visualize*. David R Hamilton PhD. https://drdavidhamilton.com/5-reasons-why-you-should-visualize/

Hampton, D. (2019, December). *The Neuroscience of How Affirmations Help Your Mental Health*. The Best Brain Possible. https://thebestbrainpossible.com/affirmations-brain-depression-anxiety/

Hawkins, M. (2011). How does violence in media desensitize children? Livestrong .com, May.

Heider, J. (2014). *The Tao of Leadership: Lao Tzu's Tao te ching Adapted for a New Age*. Green Dragon Books.

Hendel, Hilary Jacobs (2019). Trauma treatment: What is the difference between conventional talk therapy and experiential psychotherapy. Retrieved from: https://www.hilaryjacobshendel.com/post/2019/03/31/what-is-the-difference-between -conventional-talk-psychotherapy-and-aedp-psychotherapy

Hulon, W. (2018, December 14). *American College of Psychotherapy*. https://acpsy .org/dr-bessel-van-der-kolk/

Ivey, A. E., Ivey, M. B., & Zalaquett, C. P. (2013). *Intentional Interviewing and Counseling: Facilitating Client Development in a Multicultural Society*. Cengage Learning.

Ivey, A. E., Ivey, M. B., Zalaquett, C., & Quirk, K. (2009). Counseling and neuroscience: The cutting edge of the coming decade. *Counseling Today*, *52*(6), 44–48. https://ct.counseling.org/2009/12/reader-viewpoint-counseling-and-neuroscience -the-cutting-edge-of-the-coming-decade/

Jacques, M. (2004). The death of intimacy. *The Guardian*, September 18.

Jain, S., & Rubino, A. (2012). The effectiveness of emotional freedom techniques for optimal test performance. *Energy Psychology Theory, Research, & Treatment*, *4*(2), 15–26.

Jindani, F. A., & Khalsa, G. F. S. (2015). A yoga intervention program for patients suffering from symptoms of posttraumatic stress disorder: A qualitative descriptive study. *The Journal of Alternative and Complementary Medicine*, *21*(7), 401–408.

Kabat-Zinn, J. (2003). Mindfulness-based interventions in context: Past, present, and future. *Clinical Psychology: Science and Practice, 10*(2), 144–156.

Kathirasan, K. (2018). The role of mindfulness in treating addictive disorders and rehabilitation. *International Journal of Psychology and Behavior Analysis*, *4*(2). doi: 10.15344/2455-3867/2018/155

Khalsa, S. P. K. (n.d.). *Kundalini Yoga and Yogi Bhajan*. Yoga Technology. https://www.yogatech.com/Kundalini_Yoga_and_Yogi_Bhajan

Koch, S. C., Caldwell, C., & Fuchs, T. (2013). On body memory and embodied therapy. *Body, Movement and Dance in Psychotherapy*, *8*(2), 82–94.

Kornfeld, J. (1994). *Buddha's Little Instruction Book*. Barnes & Noble.

Krakow, B., Melendrez, D., Warner, T. D., Clark, J. O., Sisley, B. N., Dorin, R., ... & Hollifield, M. (2006). Signs and symptoms of sleep-disordered breathing in trauma survivors: a matched comparison with classic sleep apnea patients. *The Journal of Nervous and Mental Disease*, *194*(6), 433–439.

Lanius, Ruth & Buczynski, Ruth (n.d.). *Treating Trauma Master Series How Trauma Impacts the Major Brain Networks (and How This Affects Our Clients)* [video transcript]. National Institute for the Clinical Application of Behavioral Medicine. https://www.nicabm.com/program/treating-trauma-master/

Lazarus, C. (2016, January 26). *Can Visualization Techniques Treat Serious Diseases?* Psychology Today. https://www.psychologytoday.com/ca/blog/think -well/201601/can-visualization-techniques-treat-serious-diseases

Lazarus, C. N. (2016, January 26). Can visualization techniques treat serious diseases? *Psychology Today.* https://www.psychologytoday.com/ca/blog/think-well /201601/can-visualization-techniques-treat-serious-diseases

Levine, P. A., & Frederick, A. (1997). *Waking the Tiger: Healing Trauma: The Innate Capacity to Transform Overwhelming Experiences.* North Atlantic Books.

Ma, X., Yue, Z. Q., Gong, Z. Q., Zhang, H., Duan, N. Y., Shi, Y. T., ... & Li, Y. F. (2017). The effect of diaphragmatic breathing on attention, negative affect and stress in healthy adults. *Frontiers in Psychology, 8,* 874.

McGilchrist, I. (2019). *The Master and His Emissary.* New Haven and London: Yale University Press.

Menakem, R. (2017). *My Grandmother's Hands.* Las Vegas : Central Recovery Press.

Miller, H. (1945). *The air-conditioned Nightmare.* New York : New Directions.

Moane, Geraldine. (1999). *Gender and Colonialism : A Psychological Analysis of Oppression and Liberation.* New York: St Martin's Press.

Mullaly, B. & West, J. (2018). *Challenging Oppression and Confronting Privelege.* Oxford University Press.

NICABM (n.d). How Limbic System Therapy Can help resolve trauma [Video] Bessel Van De Kolk. https://www.nicabm.com/trauma-how-limbic-system-therapy -can-help-resolve-trauma/

NICAMB (n.d.). The Treating Trauma Master Series: A 5-Module Series on the Treatment of Trauma [video]. National Institute for the Clinical Application of Behavioral Medicine. https://www.nicabm.com/program/treating-trauma- master/

Ogden, P., Minton, K., & Pain, C. (2006). *Trauma and the Body: A Sensorimotor Approach to Psychotherapy (Norton Series on Interpersonal Neurobiology).* W.W. Norton & Company.

On the virtues of slowness. (2012). *Politics of the Hap,* January 4. Blog on the virtues of slowness.

Ortner, Jessica (2021). *Jessica Ortner's Stress Relief Audios – Free Download.* [video transcript]. The Tapping Solution. https://www.thetappingsolution.com/jessica -ortners-stress-relief-audios-free-download/

Payne, P., Levine, P. A., & Crane-Godreau, M. A. (2015). Somatic experiencing: using interoception and proprioception as core elements of trauma therapy. *Frontiers in psychology, 6,* 93.

Postman, N. (1985). Introduction. In *Amusing Ourselves to Death: Public Discourse in the Age of Show Business.* New York: Penguin.

Quiros, L., Varghese, R., & Vanidestine, T. (2020). Disrupting the single story: Challenging dominant trauma narratives through a critical race lens. *Traumatology*, *26*(2), 160–168. doi: 10.1037/trm0000223

Ross, S. (2018, January 3). *Resourcing, Pendulation and Titration: Practices from Somatic Experiencing.* https://sarahrossphd.com/resourcing-pendulation-titration -practices-somatic-experiencing/

Rothschild, B. (2017). *Autonomic Nervous System: Precision Regulation. The Body Remembers,* Volume 2: *Revolutionizing Trauma Treatment.* W.W. Norton & Company.

Rothschild, B. (2021). *Revolutionizing Trauma Treatment. Stabilization, Safety & Nervous System Balance.* W.W. Norton & Company.

Schore, A. N. (2001). The effects of early relational trauma on right brain development, affect regulation, and infant mental health. *Infant Mental Health Journal: Official Publication of The World Association for Infant Mental Health*, *22*(1–2), 201–269.

Schore, A. N. (2014). The right brain is dominant in psychotherapy. *Psychotherapy*, *51*(3), 388.

Sezgin, N., Ozcan, B., & Church, D. (2009). The effect of two psychophysiological techniques (progressive muscular relaxation and emotional freedom techniques) on test anxiety in high school students: A randomized blind controlled study. *International Journal of Healing and Caring*, *9*(1), 30–36.

Shannahoff-Khalsa, D. (1991). Lateralized rhythms of the central and autonomic nervous systems. *International Journal of Psychophysiology*, *11*(3), 225–251.

Shannahoff-Khalsa, D. S. (2005). Patient perspectives: Kundalini yoga meditation techniques for psycho-oncology and as potential therapies for cancer. *Integrative Cancer Therapies*, *4*(1), 87–100.

Shore, A. (2014). Art therapy, attachment, and the divided brain. *Art Therapy, 31*(2), 91–94.

Siegel, D. J. (2010). *The Mindful Therapist: A Clinician's Guide to Mindsight and Neural Integration (Norton Series on Interpersonal Neurobiology).* W.W. Norton & Company.

Siegel, D. J. (2015). *The Developing Mind: How Relationships and the Brain Interact to Shape Who We Are.* Guilford Publications.

Spinazzola, J., & Wilson, K. (n.d.). *Path to Recovery: Top-Down, Bottom-Up, or through the Side Door?*

Some, M. P. (1993). *Ritual: Power, Healing and Community.* New York: Penguin Compass.

Stern, D. (1985). The interpersonal world of the infant. New York: Basic Book.

Swart, T. (2019, May 9). This is a visualization exercise that actually works, according to neuroscience. *Fast Company.* https://www.fastcompany.com/90346545 /this-is-a-visualization-exercise-that-actually-works-according-to-neuroscience

Uğurbil, K. (2012). Development of functional imaging in the human brain (fMRI); the University of Minnesota experience. *Neuroimage*, *62*(2), 613–619.

Upledger Institute International Inc. (n.d.). *CST FAQs.* Upledger Institute International. https://www.upledger.com/therapies/faq.php

Van der Kolk, B. A. (2015). *The Body Keeps the Score: Brain, Mind, and Body in the Healing of Trauma.* Penguin Books.

Yalom, I. D., & Crouch, E. C. (1990). The theory and practice of group psychotherapy. *The British Journal of Psychiatry, 157*(2), 304–306.

Walker, L. E. A. (2017). Trauma practice: Historical overview. In S. N. Gold (ed.), *APA Handbook of Trauma Psychology: Trauma Practice* (pp. 1–27). American Psychological Association.

White, B. (2011, March 14). *Thought Field Therapy (TFT): "Tapping" Out Mood & Anxiety Woes?* Chipur. https://chipur.com/thought-field-therapy-tft-tapping-out-mood-and-anxiety-woes/

Winne, L. C., & Singer, M. T. (1963). Thought disorder and family relations of schizophrenics. *Archives of General Psychiatry, 1*, 9–191.

Wise, S., & Nash, E. (2013). Metaphor as heroic mediator: Imagination, creative arts therapy, and group process as agents of healing with veterans. In R. M. Scurfield & K. T. Platoni (Eds.) *Healing War Trauma: A Handbook of Creative Approaches,* (pp. 99–114). Routledge.

Index

Note: Italic page numbers refer to figures.

About The Author

Alyson Quinn has been an adjunct professor at UBC School of Social Work for seven years and taught in the Department of Educational and Counselling Psychology in the Fall term of 2019. She has been a counselor for thirty years specializing in group therapy, trauma therapy, and conflict resolution. She is a clinical counselor with a master's degree from the University of British Columbia and a diploma in conflict resolution from Royal Roads University. Alyson has taught students in a trauma informed counseling class, in a group work class, and also in Integrative Seminars, and has a great deal of experience as an individual and couple's counselor. She has authored three published books and a chapter namely *Pedagogy for an Integrative Practice* is published in the textbook, *Holistic Engagement: Transformative Social Work Education in the 21st Century*. Her textbook *Experiential Unity Theory and Model: Reclaiming Your Soul*, published in 2012, is aligned with the principles of a Trauma Informed Practice. Alyson has taught her model at both International and Canadian conferences. Alyson was born in Zimbabwe and trained as a social worker in South Africa. She launched her social work career in London, England, and then emigrated to Vancouver, Canada. Her self-help book *Reclaim Your Soul: Your Path to Healing*, published in 2014, also builds on trauma-informed principles.

Her websites are www.traumainformedpracticeinstitute.com and *alysonquinnwrites.com*